The Rainforest Medicinal Plant Guide Series

HIBISCUS FLOWER

("Roselle" *Hibiscus sabdariffa*)

NATURE'S SECRET
FOR A **HEALTHY HEART**

LESLIE TAYLOR, ND

Bestselling Author of *The Healing Power of Rainforest Herbs*

Rain-Tree
Publishers

The information and advice contained in this book are based upon the research and the professional experiences of the author, and are not intended as a substitute for consulting with a healthcare professional. The publisher and author are not responsible for any adverse effects or consequences resulting from the use of any of the suggestions discussed in this book. All matters pertaining to your physical health, including your diet and supplement routine, should be supervised by a healthcare professional who can provide medical care that is tailored to meet your individual needs.

Published by
Rain-Tree Publishers
Bullard, Texas 75757
www.rain-tree.com

ISBN: 978-1-7346847-1-1

Cover and Interior Production by Gary A. Rosenberg
www.thebookcouple.com

About the Rainforest Medicinal Plant Guide Series

This book is part of Leslie Taylor's Rainforest Medicinal Plant Guide series featuring the important medicinal plants of the rainforest that she has studied and used for more than 20 years. These guides provide factual, scientific, and vital information on how to use these powerful medicinal plants effectively to improve your health.

The author sells no herbal supplements or products other than books. The books in this series do not promote any specific brands or herbal supplement products. These definitive plant guides concern the plants and their researched effective actions and uses. The information in these guides is more extensive, complete, and unbiased than natural product companies who sell these plants as supplements can provide.

More information on Leslie Taylor's background, knowledge, and experience can be found on the Rain-Tree website (www.rain-tree.com/author.htm) See the Rain-Tree Publishers book page (www.rain-tree.com/books.htm) to learn when new plant guides in the series are released.

To my life-partner, Bob,
who trusted me with his heart—
for his heart health and for love.

Contents

Introduction

Roselle is the common name for a tropical shrub in the *Hibiscus* plant family with a scientific name of *Hibiscus sabdariffa*. When the shrub's flowers are harvested for use as a natural remedy, it is most commonly called hibiscus flowers. However, it is really the fleshy part of the flower that grows behind the petals (called a calyx) that is harvested, dried, and used in herbal supplements and remedies.

I have been researching, documenting, and writing about rainforest medicinal plants since 1995, and I must say, I rarely see a plant with so many human studies performed as have been conducted on hibiscus flowers. It is really unusual to see expensive human studies funded on a natural herbal remedy that cannot be patented and profited on by a single organization in hopes of recouping their research investment. Hibiscus flower is certainly the exception with dozens of human studies now validating its beneficial uses.

Human studies now confirm that hibiscus flowers can help lower cholesterol and blood pressure levels, and prevent clogged arteries without any of the side effects of the usual pharmaceutical drugs that treat these conditions. In fact, many people have used hibiscus flowers for these purposes in Latin America and Africa for many years, and this new research is simply confirming these traditional uses.

As a naturopath, I have used hibiscus flowers in my practice for more than 20 years to help people address high blood pressure and high cholesterol as well as clogged arteries and to improve heart function after a heart attack. It was the first natural remedy I turned to and relied on for these heart conditions. Although I have retired from my naturopathic practice, I still recommend hibiscus flowers to friends and family, including my husband, who no longer takes a statin drug or two out of three high blood pressure drugs he used to take. He's been drinking this tasty flower tea daily for the last five years, and I grow roselle in my garden for him. His cardiologist doesn't really want to know what he's doing or taking, but at each annual checkup, the doctor just says, "Whatever you're doing, keep doing it—everything looks great."

Also included in this book is new information on how natural antioxidants, like those found in hibiscus flowers, are playing important roles to help prevent arterial plaque, clogged arteries, and lower blood pressure as well as keep the heart healthy and prevent heart disease. These same antioxidants are now clinically validated to promote healthy aging and prevent many of the chronic diseases and conditions associated with aging. They have also been shown to prevent and/or improve diabetes, obesity, and many other conditions, which will be discussed in this book.

Hibiscus flowers are a popular herbal remedy for all these conditions as well as others around the world, yet most Americans know very little about the plant or how to use it, and they are unaware of the hundreds of research studies validating its many benefits. Metric tons of hibiscus flowers are now being shipped into Europe for use in natural products because information about the heart-healthy benefits of hibiscus flower and the new research on it have been shared effectively in the European natural products industry.

It's time to tell Americans how they can benefit from using this powerful natural remedy, and more important, how to use it effectively to improve their heart function and overall health. I hope the information in this book will help you discover the many effective uses of this wonderfully healthy flower and provide the hard-to-find information you need to find a good product, and take it in proper amounts.

CHAPTER 1

What Is Hibiscus?

Hibiscus is a genus of flowering plants that comprises several hundred species that grow in the tropics, subtropics, and other warm temperate climates. *Hibiscus sabdariffa* is one such species, and its common name is roselle.

Unlike its ornamental relatives, roselle's flowers are harvested and used in traditional medicine systems in many different countries. In the United States, roselle's flowers are sold as a natural herbal remedy called hibiscus flowers and sometimes simply roselle. The plant has many other common names in other countries depending on where it's grown or sold, including ambasthika, bisap, Florida cranberry, gongura, Indian sorrel, jamaica, Jamaican sorrel, karkareeh, lemon bush, oseille de Guinée, quiabo-róseo, red-sorrel, rosa de Jamaica, rosela, serení, sorrel, sour tea, and zobo.

Whatever name it is called by, roselle is a beautiful erect shrub that grows to a height of about 8 feet (2.4 meters) with many stems and branches that are dark red in color. The shrub sports medium-sized green leaves with red veins. The flower of this particular shrub is much smaller than most of the tropical hibiscus plants cultivated as ornamental plants. The flower petals can be pink or yellow, and they grow out of a fleshy ruby-red calyx right behind the flower petals. When the flowers are spent and the petals fall, the calyx is left behind, which is just as pretty as the original flower. This red calyx is what is referred to as "hibiscus flower" when it is sold or used as a natural remedy product. The calyx has also been referred to as the "fruit" of a hibiscus plant.

Roselle is thought to be native to areas from India to Malaysia, where it is commonly cultivated and thought to have been carried at an early date to Africa. However, American anthropologist G. P. Murdock published a book in 1959 on African cultures that reported roselle was domesticated by the populations of the Western Sudan (Africa) sometime before 4,000 BC. In any event, roselle has been widely distributed and cultivated in the tropics and subtropics of both hemispheres for centuries. In many areas of the West Indies and Central America, it has become naturalized and is found growing wild. Seeds are said to have been brought to the New World by enslaved Africans. Roselle was grown in Brazil as a food and for medicine in the seventeenth century and in Jamaica in the early eighteenth century. The plant was recorded being cultivated for food use in Guatemala before 1840.

Roselle can be cultivated in some areas in the Southern United States as an ornamental and medicinal plant, including in Florida and Texas, as well as in California. It needs a long growing season and is very sensitive to frost, so most in the United States grow it as an annual shrub unless they live far enough south to be completely frost-free. The shrub grows quite quickly, attaining the height of six feet or more in just six months. Live roselle plants and seeds are available to purchase in the United States for people to grow in their own backyards, and it makes a striking impact in the landscape with its many bright-red stems and pretty flowers. When sold for planting or cultivating here in the United States, it is often referred to as Florida cranberry or just roselle to help distinguish it from the many different hibiscus ornamental plants that are sold for their beautiful and much larger flowers (but don't have any medicinal value).

Roselle leaves are edible, taste very lemony with a slightly bitter bite, and are often used to prepare "sour soup" or sprinkled in salads for a lemony punch. The leaves taste much like the European lemony sorrel herb widely grown as a vegetable and seasoning, which is why roselle is sometimes called sorrel, red sorrel, or Jamaican sorrel.

It is the fleshy flower calyx, however, that is used to prepare a popular beverage in many countries and used medicinally. A tea is prepared with the calyces that tastes very much like cranberry juice and is usually sweetened to improve the tart taste. It is drunk either hot or iced. This bright red "juice" of the calyces that is released into the tea has even been turned into wine, jelly and jam, sauces, and syrups. The flowers contain pectin, the natural substance needed to thicken or "jell" jellies and jams. Very little added pectin is necessary to make a good jelly with the flower calyces.

Traditional Uses in Herbal Medicine

All parts of the roselle shrub have been used medicinally around the world: leaves, flower calyces, seeds, and seed oil. This book focuses on the uses of roselle's calyces or, as commonly called, hibiscus flowers. The rule of thumb in most traditional medicine systems is to prepare a decoction (gently boiling or simmering the flowers in water for 10 minutes) if you're using dried flower calyces and to prepare an infusion with the fresh flower calyces (pour boiling water over the fresh calyces and let steep for 10 minutes). More specific information on preparing your own flower remedies is provided in the Consumer Guide on page 71.

In Brazilian traditional medicine systems, hibiscus flower tea is used for anxiety, heart conditions, flu, fast heart rate, kidney disorders, colic, diarrhea, uterine pain, inflammation, labyrinthitis (an inner ear disorder), snakebite, and pneumonia. Over the last several years, cultivation of roselle has increased in Brazil as it is now being widely used as a weight-loss aid as well as an herbal remedy for high cholesterol and high blood pressure. The hibiscus flower iced drink is considered cooling and is used for heatstroke. It is often given to tourists unused to the humid, hot tropics, and sometimes it is even employed to cool down a fever.

In India, hibiscus flowers are used in traditional medicine as a diuretic; as a mild laxative; for the treatment of kidney, heart, and liver diseases; for high blood pressure; and for feverous conditions and skin inflammations. The flower tea is used by the Zeliang tribe in Northeast India to treat stomach disorders, as a blood-purifying agent, and as a hair tonic. In Jharkhand, in Eastern India, hibiscus flower tea is recommended for curing coughs, colds, and malaria. The flower tea is used by the tribes of Maharashtra in Western India and the Karbis tribe in Northeast India as a general antidote for food and chemical poisoning. Hibiscus flowers are used for treating stomachaches and digestion problems, hemorrhoids, and menstrual and other gynecological disorders by tribes of Andaman and Nicobar Islands, India.

In African herbal medicine systems, hibiscus flowers are used for their antimicrobial, emollient (softening and soothing), fever-reducing, diuretic, vermifuge (worm-expelling), and sedative properties. In Nigeria, Sudan, Iran, and other countries, the flower tea is used to lower blood pressure, to treat other heart conditions, and as a diuretic. In many African countries, beverages made from hibiscus flowers provide relief during hot weather by increasing the flow of blood to the skin surface and dilating the pores to cool the skin. The flower tea also is used widely in Egypt for the treatment of heart and nerve diseases.

In Mexico, roselle is called jamaica (pronounced *ha-MY-ka*), and the flower tea is a very popular beverage, widely sold and drunk throughout the country. It has long been used as a high blood pressure and heart tonic herbal remedy, as a weight-loss aid, as a cooling beverage to combat heat and humidity, and for various infections, including tuberculosis, foodborne bacteria, and fungi/candida. It's also touted as a respected morning-after remedy for hangovers in Mexico and Guatemala. Dried and/or fresh hibiscus flowers can be found in most grocery stores and street markets in Mexico and other Latin American countries as it's quite popular.

ETHNIC MEDICINAL USES OF HIBISCUS FLOWERS	
Africa	For anemia, bacterial infections, coughs, diabetes, diarrhea, fever, genital problems, heart conditions, high cholesterol, hypertension, inflammation, intestinal worms, kidney stones, malaria, parasites, respiratory infections, skin rashes and conditions, sore throat, tuberculosis, viral infections, urinary tract infections, weight loss, and wounds; to lower body temperature; to increase urination, bowel function, and the secretion of bile in the liver
Brazil	For anxiety, cavities, colic, diarrhea, ear infections and disorders, fever, flu, gum disease, heart conditions, heatstroke, high blood pressure, high cholesterol, inflammation, kidney disorders and infections, kidney stones, inflammation, obesity, pneumonia, snakebite, tachycardia, tuberculosis, urinary infections, and uterine pain
Egypt	For bacterial infections, candida, cardiac and nerve diseases, diarrhea, hypertension, high cholesterol, respiratory tract infections, urinary tract infections, and weight loss; to increase urination and lower body temperature

Europe	For bacterial infections, foodborne bacteria and food poisoning, high cholesterol, hypertension, and weight loss
Greece	For high cholesterol, hypertension, infections, and weight loss
Guatemala	For anemia, diabetes, gum disease, hangover, heatstroke, high cholesterol, hypertension, infections, and weight loss
India	For colds, cough, dyspnea (difficulty in breathing), fever, food poisoning, gynecological disorders, heart diseases, hemorrhoids, hypertension, hair loss, infections, kidney stones, kidney disorders, liver diseases, malaria, menstrual disorders, obesity, skin disorders, upset stomach, and stomach disorders; as a mild laxative and restorative tonic; to increase urination, bowel function, and the secretion of bile in the liver
Mexico	For anemia, diabetes, hangover, high cholesterol, hypertension, kidney stones, and weight loss; to increase urination, bowel function, and the secretion of bile in the liver
Sudan	For aiding digestion, colds, clearing sinuses, clearing mucus, hypertension, promoting kidney function, and reducing fever; as a general tonic and diuretic
Elsewhere	For bacterial infections, food poisoning, high blood pressure, high cholesterol, liver disorders, malaria, and parasitic infections; to lower body temperature and increase urination

In Europe, much of the new research on hibiscus flowers is being disseminated in the European natural products market. This has fueled new herbal supplements as natural products for high blood pressure, high cholesterol, and weight loss. In fact, these newly validated uses have been much more widely disseminated around the world much more effectively than here in the United States.

Hibiscus flowers are now used as herbal remedies for the treatment of various cardiovascular risk factors, including hypertension (in Egypt, Jordan, Trinidad, and Tobago), for high blood pressure (in Jordan and Iraq), for high cholesterol (in Jordan, Greece, Brazil, Trinidad, and Tobago), and for obesity (in Iraq, Greece, and Brazil). People in Mexico have been using hibiscus flowers for all four of these conditions for more than 50 years, and it was the traditional uses in Mexico that fueled much of the subsequent research discussed in the next chapter.

Plant Chemicals in Hibiscus Flowers

Hibiscus flowers contain a host of beneficial chemicals that are mostly classified as polysaccharides, anthocyanins, flavonoids, and polyphenols. The flower calyces are best known for being a very good source of important antioxidant chemicals called anthocyanins. Antioxidants fight free radicals and reactive oxygen species (ROS), as well as relieve oxidative stress and cellular damage from these oxidizing agents.

Anthocyanidins are well-studied antioxidant chemicals that naturally occur in medicinal plants and berries with known biological activities. Delphinidin 3-sambubioside and cyanidin 3-sambubioside have been reported to be the anthocyanins in the greatest amount in hibiscus flowers and cyanidin 3-O-rutinoside, delphinidin 3-O-glucoside, and cyanidin 3,5-diglucoside are present in lower amounts.

Hibiscus flowers also contain a significant amount of phenolic acids, including protocatechuic acid and hibiscus acid, with lesser amounts of well-known polyphenol chemicals, including chlorogenic acid, quercetin, caffeic acid, catechin, gallocatechins, and gallocatechin gallates.

Polyphenol chemicals have been associated with beneficial effects on human health, such as reducing the risk of various diseases like cancer, diabetes, obesity, and cardiovascular and brain diseases. Polyphenols are well documented to provide therapeutic actions in low dosages. To date, 37 different polyphenolic chemicals have been identified in hibiscus flowers. In addition, hibiscus flowers are a good source of flavonoids with the main ones being gossypetin, hibiscetin, and sabdaretine. Some of these are novel plant chemicals, found only in hibiscus flowers.

Roselle's chemical composition has shown that the therapeutic potency of the flowers could be traced to the presence of bioactive compounds. Bioactive compounds such as flavonoids (quercetin, luteolin, and others); chlorogenic acid, gossypetin, hibiscetin, phenols, some phenolic acids including a significant amount of hibiscus acid; and anthocyanins such as delphinidin 3 sambubioside and cyanidin 3 sambubioside were detected as the main active ingredients in the water extract or tea of the flowers. These bioactive compounds together or alone have been reported in many studies to possess potent antioxidant, anti-inflammatory, and anticancer effects and may also help control diabetes, as well as prevent cardiovascular disease and obesity.

The food value of hibiscus flowers indicates that they are a great source of fiber (including resistant fiber that acts as a prebiotic to encourage the growth of beneficial bacteria in the gut), calcium, phosphorus, and protein and provides other essential nutrients as well. The flowers contain a large amount of pectin. Fruit pectin has shown cholesterol-lowering actions in several studies. The fat content of the flowers deliver numerous fatty acids, including beneficial omega-3 fatty acids, and researchers have reported that some of these fatty acids contribute to the flower's antibacterial, anti-inflammatory, and antioxidant actions.

FOOD VALUE OF HIBISCUS FLOWERS (PER 100 G FRESH/10 G DRIED)	
Protein	1.145 g
Fat	2.61 g
Fiber	12.0 g
Calcium	1263 mg
Phosphorus	273.2 mg
Iron	8.98 mg
Carotene	0.029 mg
Thiamine	0.117 mg
Riboflavin	0.277 mg
Niacin	3.765 mg
Ascorbic acid	6.7 mg

The plant chemistry of hibiscus flowers is a perfect example of nature's synergy in a medicinal plant. While many of the individual polyphenol, flavonoid, and anthocyanin chemicals are the subject of research to determine their individual actions and benefits, researchers have noted repeatedly that there is a synergy, or additive effect, of these chemicals working together. The actions and benefits of hibiscus flower tea, which contains all the chemicals working together synergistically, is reported in many studies to be much greater than the action of any isolated single chemical.

Much of the new research detailed in the next chapter simply studied hibiscus flower tea as a whole and researchers rarely attributed the beneficial actions they were observing to any single chemical due to this plant's well-documented synergy and many active beneficial chemicals. This is rather unusual for plant research in general, but most plant research in the United States is funded by drug companies looking for novel plant chemicals with beneficial actions they can turn into profitable new drugs. Once they target a chemical or two in a plant they're studying, all the focus and research shifts to the targeted chemicals rather than the whole plant they found the chemical in. However, in the case of roselle, the dramatic results of the natural flower tea (with its many chemicals working together) kept fueling research on the flower tea as a whole instead of any single plant chemical it contains.

The chemicals identified in hibiscus flowers thus far include the following: 2-o-trans-caffeoyl-hydroxycitric acid,

3-caffeoylquinic acid, 4-caffeoylquinic acid, 5-caffeoylqui-
nic acid, 5-hydroxymethylfurfural, 5-O-caffeoylshikimic
acid, arabinose, caffeic acid, caffeoylquinic acid isomers,
catechin, chlorogenic acid, chlorogenic acid isomers, citric acid, coumaroylquinic acid, cyanidin-3-sambubioside,
cyanidin-3,5-diglucoside, delphinidin, delphinidin-3-sam-
bubioside, ellagic acid, eugenol, feruloyl, feruloyl quinic
acid derivatives, ergosterol, gallic acid, gallocatechin, gallocatechin gallate, galloyl ester, galacturonic acid, glucu-
ronic acid, gossypitrin, gossytrin, gossypetin glucosides,
hibiscitrin, hibiscetin-3-glucoside, hibiscus acid, hibiscus
acid 6-methyl ester, hibiscus acid glucoside, hydroxycitric acids, kaempferol, kaempferol-3-glucoside, kae-
mpferol-3-o-rutinoside, kaempferol-3-o-sambubioside,
kaempferol-3-p-coumaryl-glucoside, luteolin, malic
acid, mannose, methyl gallate, methyl-epigallocatechin,
myricetin, myricetin-3-arabinogalactoside, n-feruloyltyr-
amide, pectin, pelargonidin, pelargonic acid, protocatechuic acid, protocatechuic acid glucosides, quercetin,
quercetin derivatives, quercetin-3-glucoside, querce-
tin-3-rutinoside, quercetin-3-sambioside, rhamnose, β-sit-
osterol, sabdaretin, sabdaritrin, sambubioside, tartaric
acid, tiliroside, and xylose.

CHAPTER 2

The Heart-Healthy Benefits of Hibiscus Flowers

This chapter provides information on the research and clinical studies conducted on hibiscus flowers. More than 450 studies have been published thus far, and this natural remedy is the subject of ongoing research in many areas. Most research on hibiscus flower has been performed outside the United States, in countries that are much more open to herbal remedies and herbal drugs. These developing nations fund research looking for effective, low-cost therapies for common diseases and ailments to improve people's health and lower their healthcare costs rather than patenting and selling high-cost prescription drugs. This research includes human studies and full human clinical trials, which are rare for a natural herbal remedy that no single company can patent and profit from.

The exciting news is that human studies now confirm that hibiscus flowers can treat high cholesterol, high blood pressure, clogged arteries, and heart disease. Based on a large body of research conducted around the world over the last 10 years, we now know that chronic inflammation and oxidative stress are playing a significant role in the development and progression of all these conditions, as well as quite a few others. Hibiscus flower's positive effect on high cholesterol, high blood pressure, clogged arteries, and heart diseases are, in part, due to the ability of the flowers to address and relieve chronic inflammation and oxidative stress effectively, so let's begin the discussion there.

Antioxidant Actions: Fight Free Radicals & Relieve Oxidative Stress

The first area of research on hibiscus flowers is one of the most documented and verified—the antioxidant action of hibiscus flowers. Many people understand that antioxidants "fights free radicals," but most don't realize that antioxidants can work in four different ways. Substances called free radicals, and particularly a group of free radicals called reactive oxygen species (ROS), are a product of normal life, created by metabolizing foods and various other chemical interactions in our bodies, which are quite normal.

Our bodies have a natural built-in system that is supposed to keep ROS in check and at healthy levels. This includes natural chemicals we produce in our bodies called antioxidants, and they are capable of scavenging or deactivating ROS. However, many diseases, health conditions, and internal deregulations can occur that greatly increases ROS, which can then overwhelm or disable our natural antioxidant system. Other things can limit our ability to produce these antioxidants. For example, just eating too much sugar (especially high-fructose corn syrup, which is found in soda) reduces our bodies' ability to produce our own natural antioxidant chemicals to keep ROS at healthy levels. If we produce too much ROS or our natural antioxidant system becomes overwhelmed or fails, the result is oxidative stress.

Oxidative stress can damage many different types of cells and organs. ROS and free radicals are particularly damaging to the cells in the heart and cardiovascular system because they are actually circulating in our bloodstream. Thousands of studies report the mechanisms by which ROS can contribute to the development of clogged arteries, high blood pressure, peripheral vascular disease, coronary artery disease, cardiomyopathy, heart failure, and cardiac arrhythmias.

When cells suffer oxidative stress, inflammation results, and left untreated, even more cellular damage occurs. When oxidative stress begins to damage cells, the immune system gets triggered to repair or remove the damaged cells, and this results in even more inflammation as well as the generation of even more ROS, which creates a vicious circle. Inflammation is a natural process our immune system uses to repair or eliminate unhealthy cells. Therefore, oxidative stress usually goes hand in hand with inflammation, and it can result in a chronic low-level state of inflammation throughout our bodies.

This can negatively impact various organs and internal processes. If you have never heard of ROS, free radicals, and/or antioxidants before, you might find another book in Rainforest Medicinal Plant Guide Series very helpful: *Acerola – Nature's Secret to Fight Free Radicals*. It explains how natural plant antioxidants react with free radicals and ROS to relieve oxidative stress and chronic inflammation in much greater detail. See Amazon.com or the Raintree website for more information on how to obtain the book.

Tens of thousands of research studies have been published on chronic inflammation and oxidative stress and the roles they play in numerous diseases. We now know that inflammation and oxidative stress can be a cause or a contributing factor to a wide range of diseases, including almost every chronic disease. From heart diseases, diabetes, Alzheimer's disease, and cancer to high cholesterol levels, autoimmune diseases, and even obesity—chronic inflammation and oxidative stress are playing significant roles. The amount and type of inflammation in our bodies also helps determine how well or poorly we age.

Taking antioxidants to treat and interrupt this oxidative process is well known to be beneficial in numerous conditions where ROS is damaging cells, but picking the right antioxidant is necessary. Not all antioxidants work the same way, and there are different types and species of ROS that require different methods to address them. That's where the synergy of a plant like roselle shines.

Hibiscus flowers contains over 20 strong antioxidant

natural plant compounds that employ four different methods to address damaging ROS. The main natural chemicals found in the flowers with well-established antioxidant actions include protocatechuic acid, anthocyanins, quercetin, catechins, and polyphenols, which have been shown to protect cellular components from damage by oxidation. This makes the flower tea a great natural antioxidant remedy with enormous benefits in numerous conditions where oxidative stress and damage is an issue.

Hibiscus flower's strong antioxidant actions are now well accepted and established in human, animal, and test-tube research. A flower tea was first reported with anti-oxidant actions in 2004 and, since that time, more than 40 other studies have been published reporting and con-firming the flower's effective and beneficial antioxidant actions. These studies included *in vitro* studies (intro-ducing flower teas to various oxidative chemicals in test tubes), numerous animal studies, and four human stud-ies. (See the reference section for a listing of these studies.)

Human Antioxidant Studies

It is well known that strenuous exercise promotes the generation of ROS and oxidative stress. Researchers in Iran gave 54 male soccer players hibiscus flower tea and reported in their 2017 study that it provided antioxidant actions and it had: "beneficial effects on oxidative stress status in male athletes." In 2016, medical researchers in Mexico gave 17 patients with Marfan syndrome (a heart disease that results in significant oxidative stress to the heart) a hibiscus flower tea. They reported that hibiscus flowers provided great benefits in reducing their oxidative stress levels. In 2012, German researchers measured the antioxidant actions of hibiscus flowers in healthy volunteers and also reported that it significantly reduced the oxidative stress markers in their blood through the hibiscus flower's antioxidant actions.

Lowering oxidative stress in our bodies can provide many health benefits, and it can provide therapeutic effects in numerous diseases and conditions where oxidative stress is playing a significant role, especially in the heart. However, the research reveals even more. Hibiscus flower can not only reduce free radicals and reduce oxidative stress, it can also repair the damage that ROS has already caused.

Cellular-Protective Actions:
Protect Your Heart, Brain, Kidneys, and Liver

Common antioxidants, especially the vitamin kind of antioxidants (vitamin A, C, and E) and those produced naturally by our bodies (enzymes named superoxide dismutase, glutathione peroxidase, glutathione reductase, and catalases), are well documented to be able to protect cells from ROS by "quenching" free radicals. Free radicals are reactive/unstable because they are missing an electron. By lending free radicals an extra electron, this stops them from doing more damage and renders them into stable molecules instead of reactive ones. Strong plant antioxidants, including the antioxidants in hibiscus flowers, can also neutralize these free radicals and ROS in the same manner, and they have been shown to relieve oxidative stress in three additional ways.

In addition to lending electrons, plant antioxidants can also suppress the formation of ROS by inhibiting certain enzymes involved in their production; therefore, fewer ROS are actually created. The third method employed is the ability to trigger or increase the body's natural production of antioxidants and send them to cells under oxidative stress. Much like an injury signals the immune system to send healing agents to the site of an injury, plant antioxidants can signal the built-in antioxidant system to send its healing antioxidants to the site of oxidative stress in the body and encourage the body to produce more of them.

Lastly, we have various metals in our bodies (including the iron circulating in our blood), which can become oxidized and damage cells, much like ROS does. Some strong plant antioxidants, like those found in hibiscus flowers, are capable of interacting with oxidized metals and converting metal pro-oxidants in the body into stable products, much like they stabilize or neutralize free radicals, which reduces oxidative stress.

When a substance can address ROS and the oxidative stress created by ROS in all four antioxidant methods, you typically have what is called a cellular-protective antioxidant. In addition to the 42 regular antioxidant studies, a host of other studies have been published on hibiscus flower's cellular-protective abilities for numerous different organs that are known to be damaged by oxidative stress. These cellular-protective antioxidant natural compounds can actually prevent the damage normally caused by ROS and/or in some instances, can help repair or restore function to cells already damaged by oxidative stress.

Thus far, 12 animal studies and one human study report that hibiscus flower tea can help protect the heart from known factors which creates oxidative stress and damage to the heart and in the cardiovascular system. Moreover, 18 different animal studies report that hibiscus flowers can protect the liver from oxidative stress created by various chemicals, toxins, drugs, and diseases that normally damage the liver. Three of these studies reported that a flower tea reversed some of the induced liver damage in the test subjects. Nine more studies reported hibiscus flowers had the ability to protect the kidneys and renal system, and six studies revealed the flowers protected the brain from oxidative stress. Other studies reported that hibiscus flowers could also protect the pancreas from oxidative stress, which is well established to occur in people with diabetes (there is more on this later).

Anti-inflammatory and Immune-Modulation Actions

As you just learned, when we relieve oxidative stress with the effective natural antioxidant compounds in hibiscus flowers, we are also reducing chronic inflammation that is caused by oxidative stress. However, hibiscus flowers have been reported to relieve inflammation in other ways as well. Hibiscus flowers have been reported to have anti-inflammatory actions in 11 studies published between 1996 and 2019 by researchers around the world. Most of these studies reported these anti-inflammatory actions were coming from anthocyanins, which, as you learned earlier, is a group of natural antioxidant compounds in hibiscus flowers. Anthocyanins have been well studied over the years, and more than 400 published studies report that anthocyanins relieve inflammation in numerous ways. With the flowers delivering a significant amount of these beneficial anthocyanins (up to 50 percent of the active chemicals in hibiscus flower are anthocyanins), it's of little wonder that hibiscus flowers provide anti-inflammatory benefits.

One way of relieving inflammation is by modulating our immune response. Our immune system creates inflammation in our bodies by creating pro-inflammatory chemicals that cause inflammation. This natural process is how the immune system gets healing agents to repair injuries and fight infection at the site of injury or infection. However, when individual cells in our bodies are damaged by individual types of ROS throughout our bodies, these immune cells and pro-inflammatory chemicals are sent throughout our bodies, and it can result in chronic low-grade inflammation throughout the body. We can reduce the amount of ROS, which will certainly help; however, hibiscus flowers have been reported to cool off the immune response and reduce the number of these pro-inflammatory substances, which provides an anti-inflammatory action through the modification of the immune system.

Concerning hibiscus flowers specifically, three animal studies published in 2008 and 2017 reported that the flowers had these types of immune-modulation actions that reduced inflammation. These studies reported that the flowers inhibited an inflammatory chemical in the body named COX-2 in one study, and reduced the production other pro-inflammatory chemicals called interleukins in two other studies. One of these studies reported that the flowers increased some immune cells (natural killer cells) that fight disease-causing bacteria and bad cells while reducing other pro-inflammatory chemicals. This is not unusual for plant remedies that contain anthocyanins—this immune-modulation anti-inflammatory action was well documented in those 400-plus studies on the anti-inflammatory actions of anthocyanins.

In 2014, researchers in Spain studied a polyphenol extract of hibiscus flowers for its actions on heart function in humans and tracked inflammation factors. Their research reported that the flower tea reduced all seven of the pro-inflammatory chemicals they tested and lowered overall CRP (c-reactive protein—an inflammatory marker that helps to determine the amount of inflammation present in the body).

In a 2016 human study, doctors in Taiwan gave hibiscus flower tea to patients in a long-term care hospital who had urinary catheters and noted fewer urinary tract infections (UTI) and renal inflammation in those who took the tea over those who didn't. They then studied this effect in mice to determine how it could have provided this effect. The bacteria known to infect the urinary tract produce toxins called lipopolysaccharides (LPS), and LPS causes inflammation directly and also activates the immune system to send pro-inflammatory chemicals (called cytokines) to the site of infection. The researchers gave mice a hibiscus flower tea for seven days and then gave them an injection of LPS directly. They reported that the tea was able to stop the pro-inflammatory cytokines from infiltrating the kidney and prevented inflammation in the urinary tract. They also reported that, based on their research, they believed a hibiscus flower tea could be very beneficial for people experiencing UTIs.

Researchers in Japan studied the immune-modulating anti-inflammatory actions of one of the main anthocyanins, delphinidin 3-sambubioside, in LPS-induced inflammation in mice and *in vitro*. They reported in 2015 that this anthocyanin was capable of reducing or deactivating the inflammation produced by at least five different pro-inflammatory cytokines. In addition to hibiscus flower's anthocyanins, researchers in China have reported that other natural compounds in the flowers, called polysaccharides, also have similar immune-modulation actions. Other research reported from India and Nigeria have also confirmed hibiscus flower's immune-modulation actions, which led to reducing inflammation.

The science is pretty clear: Hibiscus flowers provide very beneficial actions to reduce inflammation, fight free radicals, reduce the production of ROS, and prevent oxidative stress. Next, you'll learn how these actions are playing significant roles in helping control cholesterol levels, prevent clogged arteries, and reduce the risk of developing cardiovascular diseases.

Reduction and Prevention of Clogged Arteries

One of the first important diseases that ROS, oxidative stress, and inflammation play a major role in is a condition called atherosclerosis. This is the medical term for the buildup of plaque that clogs arteries. To understand how hibiscus flowers prevent clogged arteries, we need to understand how the arteries get clogged in the first place—and it's *not* from just having too much cholesterol or too much "bad" cholesterol circulating in the bloodstream.

The real problem is, as we age, we create and have accumulated much more ROS in our blood, organs, and cells. When LDL cholesterol (the "bad" cholesterol) circulating in the bloodstream gets oxidized by these ROS, it gets heavier and sticky and can begin to accumulate as fatty deposits in our veins and arteries. Another ROS-like substance in our bodies, called advanced glycation end products (AGEs), also accumulates as we age. AGEs create much of the same damaging effects on cells in our bodies as ROS, especially in the heart and arteries.

Unfortunately, when AGEs damage certain types of

cells, the interaction causes even more ROS to be formed, and AGE's are well known to cause inflammation. Where AGEs go in the body and which cells they damage are mainly controlled by the cell surface receptors that signal them to migrate and accumulate there. The receptors for AGEs are present on the surface of all cells relevant to atherosclerotic processes, which is why they can be so damaging to the heart and arteries and why they are specifically linked to the promotion of arterial plaque. There's more on AGEs in chapter 3, since hibiscus flowers have shown in recent research to reduce the production of AGEs, interrupt receptors, and prevent AGEs from damaging cells.

The bottom line in arterial plaque—it just can't be formed in our bodies without ROS and/or AGEs. These ROS and AGEs are circulating in our bloodstream, putting them in constant contact with our arteries and veins, and in elevated levels, they negatively affect our health and are the main cause of clogged arteries. Normal LDL cholesterol is not the problem. It is LDL cholesterol that is oxidized by ROS and glycated by AGEs as well as the damage they do to the lining of our arteries that are the real causes of clogged arteries.

That's why clogged arteries are usually only an issue in older people—the older we are, the more ROS and AGEs we have accumulated in our bodies, which results in more damaged cholesterol that clogs our arteries. Since additional ROS and AGEs can be generated in significant amounts from external factors like smoking cigarettes, chemical and pollution exposure, and eating too much sugar, as well as internal factors like being overweight or having diabetes, clogged arteries can be experienced prior to old age. It all depends on what other factors and risks we have that elevate our ROS and AGE levels that can raise our risks of developing clogged arteries.

An important component in the progression of atherosclerosis is how the immune system reacts to the cellular damage caused by ROS and AGEs. When the immune system starts reacting to the cellular damage caused by ROS in our arteries, immune cells start infiltrating the area, causing low-grade inflammation and damage to the cells in the lining of our arteries. In addition, plaque can be perceived as a foreign invader by these immune cells whose role it is to protect us from invaders, so this triggers the immune system to respond as well. When immune cells are recruited to the site of oxidative or glycated damage in an artery or these sticky oxidized fat deposits in the artery, a new cell is created, called a foam cell. Foam cells are really just cholesterol-laden immune cells because the immune cell engulfed or "ate" an oxidized cholesterol cell just like they're supposed to engulf foreign cells such as bacteria. It is these foam cells that are the second main component or ingredient in arterial plaque.

Foam cells and other immune cells called to the region to repair ROS and AGE damage promote the growth of arterial plaque, growing it to levels to create a blockage in an artery. These immune cells, trapped in the area by interacting with foam cells and ongoing damage to the arterial wall, secrete inflammatory substances (called interleukins and tumor necrosis factor), create more ROS, and create other substances that are growth factors for other cells in the area. When these growth factors stimulate cells found in the lining of arteries (called endothelial cells), the artery wall becomes thicker from the inside, thereby narrowing the size of the artery and speeding the blockage. Medically, this is called vascular smooth muscle cell (VSMC) proliferation. When you add in the damage to cells in the lining of arteries by AGEs, the glycation causes these cells to harden and become stiffer, which is the main cause of hardened arteries.

Therefore, hibiscus flower's ability to reduce and prevent ROS and AGEs and the cellular damage they cause, prevent LDL from oxidizing, as well as reduce inflammation and immune cell activation is how hibiscus flowers prevent clogged arteries. Hibiscus flower's antioxidant, anti-inflammatory, and immune-modulating natural compounds previously discussed are playing significant roles in this process. These actions and abilities have also been confirmed with scientific research specifically studying hibiscus flower's anti-atherosclerotic actions.

Six animal studies have reported that hibiscus flowers have an anti-atherosclerotic effect. Some researchers attributed this action to reducing or eliminating oxidized LDL cholesterol, preventing or reducing foam cell formation, inhibiting smooth muscle cell proliferation (reducing thickened artery walls), and/or reducing or preventing immune cell activation and/or the inflammation and cellular damage caused by these pro-inflammatory chemicals. One of these research groups studying hibiscus flowers in rabbits noted all these effects and also reported that the flowers prevented the arterial plaque from calcifying and glycating (causing hardening of the arteries).

The active chemicals in hibiscus flowers that have been confirmed with anti-atherosclerotic actions include cyanidin 3 rutinoside, delphinidin 3 sambubioside, cyanidin 3 sambubioside, cyanidin 3 glucoside, delphinidin 3 glucoside, and hibiscus acid. All these compounds have demonstrated in research to prevent atherosclerosis through several mechanisms such as the antioxidative activity, inhibition of LDL oxidation, and smooth muscle cell proliferation. Most researchers report that these natural plant chemicals work together synergistically to provide a much greater effect than any single chemical they isolated and tested individually.

With all these positive actions, hibiscus flower is an important and effective natural remedy to prevent and reduce clogged arteries. However, if we're really treating the root causes of blocked arteries by reducing or stopping LDL cholesterol from being oxidized or glycated (which really begins the whole artery-blocking process), do we really need to lower our cholesterol levels to very low levels with statin drugs? That will be for you to decide, but the good news is: If you want to do both, an even greater amount of research has been performed on hibiscus flower's ability to lower cholesterol levels as well. These actions are discussed next.

Cholesterol-Lowering Actions

Before we discuss lowering cholesterol levels, let's review why we have cholesterol in our bodies in the first place. Cholesterol is necessary to maintain our health and the health of all our cells. Cholesterol is required to produce various essential vitamins; metabolize minerals; manufacture hormones like testosterone, estrogen, and progesterone; keep our immune system operating at optimal levels; and plays other essential roles. For example, cholesterol is an essential component of the membranes that surround all human cells. Cholesterol also functions as a powerful antioxidant, thus protecting us against cancer and aging. The brain has a higher cholesterol content than any other organ. In fact, about 25 percent of the body's cholesterol is found in the brain; it is required for the brain to function normally.

The liver makes about 80 percent of the cholesterol we need to stay healthy. Only about 20 percent comes from the foods we eat—and it's not just from so-called high-cholesterol foods. If we eat only 200 to 300 milligrams of cholesterol a day (one egg yolk has about 200 milligrams), the liver will produce an additional 800 milligrams per day from the fat, sugars, and proteins we consume.

Aside from the cholesterol consumed, for the body to produce cholesterol, a specific enzyme is required to make it. This enzyme is called HMG-CoA reductase, and it's mainly produced in the liver (smaller amounts are produced the brain). Statin drugs reduce cholesterol by interfering with or inhibiting this HMG-CoA reductase enzyme so less cholesterol is produced by the liver. Some statin drugs have the ability to cross the blood-brain barrier to reduce cholesterol in the brain, and some cannot.

Statin Drugs and Their Side Effects

Many people who take statin drugs to lower their cholesterol are well aware of the negative side effects, including fatigue, memory problems, "brain fog," muscle pain, and muscle weakness, to name just a few. What most people don't know is why.

An important substance, coenzyme Q10, is also produced in the liver, and it requires the same HMG-CoA enzyme to produce it. Also known as CoQ10, this compound helps generate energy in all our cells. Think of how gasoline fuels a car—crude oil has to be refined into gasoline first. Inside all our cells are substances called mitochondria that act as "mini-refineries." Cells take in CoQ10 as crude oil, and mitochondria refine it into another substance called ATP (adenosine triphosphate). ATP is the gasoline our cells need to fuel their cellular processes properly and even just to survive. In fact, all life on our planet depends on ATP to fuel cellular functions and sustain life.

When statin drugs do their job reducing cholesterol produced by the liver, they also simultaneously reduce the amount of CoQ10 produced by inhibiting the same enzyme required for the body's manufacture of both. In fact, most of the negative side effects of statin drugs are the result of not enough CoQ10 available to the cells. Low cellular energy from not enough CoQ10 to make ATP in muscle cells causes weakness and pain in muscles, low cellular energy in brain cells causes brain fog and memory loss, and low energy in heart cells are the main reason statin drugs fail to prevent as many cardiac events as doctors thought they would.

The lack of CoQ10 available to the heart from statin drugs is now thought to be a significant contributing factor or cause of the rising levels of heart failure we are seeing today. Deaths attributed to heart failure more than doubled in the first 10 years after statins were routinely prescribed. In addition, various animal and human studies confirm the association between a much higher risk of heart failure with statin use. Low-energy heart cells just wear out faster, and the heart is a muscle; muscles cannot work well with low CoQ10 levels decreasing ATP energy. The heart muscle is especially susceptible because it uses so much energy to operate continuously.

The whole concept of statin drugs and why they are taken is based on the assertion that excess cholesterol in the bloodstream is a key contributor to artery-clogging plaque, which can accumulate and set the stage for a heart attack. Therefore, the main reason for taking a statin drug is because it's supposed to prevent clogged arteries and prevent heart attacks. However, they are leaving out a really important and significant factor that most people who take statin drugs just don't know. As previously discussed, cholesterol isn't the problem. It's only when cholesterol becomes oxidized that it sticks to the artery walls and becomes a problem.

The Cholesterol Hypothesis Controversy

Since statin drugs do nothing to prevent oxidation, they must lower the total cholesterol, including HDL (the "good" cholesterol), to *much* lower levels, which in turn, lowers the amount of oxidized HDL cholesterol. And the lower the cholesterol levels, the lower the CoQ10 levels. However, are statins lowering cholesterol levels too low unnecessarily while ignoring the real cause of clogged arteries and other heart diseases? Quite possibly.

Research published in 2015 by an international team of researchers who performed a systematic review of studies of more than 68,000 people over age 60 raised questions about the benefits of statin drug treatments, which just lowered over all cholesterol. In fact, their research called into question the "cholesterol hypothesis," which previously suggested people with high cholesterol and especially high LDL cholesterol (LDL-C) are more at risk of dying from cardiovascular disease. These researchers reported that after age 60, higher cholesterol levels actually prolonged life. They summarized their research saying: "If LDL-C is accumulating in arteries over a lifetime to cause heart disease, then why is it that elderly people with the highest LDL-C live the longest? Since people over the age of 60 with high LDL-C live the longest, why should we lower it?"

This study obviously caused a great deal of controversy as well as criticism, although other independent researchers around the world (not connected to or performed by drug companies who sell statin drugs) have reported similar findings over the years. Beginning in the mid-2000s, researchers in Japan, China, France, Finland, and even the United States began to question this cholesterol hypothesis and the ability of statins to reduce cardiovascular risks. There are, of course, other studies (funded by drug companies that sell statin drugs) that refute these researchers' work and continue to support and validate their cholesterol hypothesis.

In one study conducted by Columbia University College of Physicians and Surgeons in New York, researchers reported in 2005 that in more than 2,000 patients over age 65, people with the lowest cholesterol levels were approximately twice as likely to die (of all causes) as those with the highest cholesterol levels. A Finnish research group reported in 2012 that they followed more than 1,200 patients over age 65 for 10 years. They reported the main risk factor for increased mortality in the population they studied was *oxidized* LDL cholesterol levels, not total cholesterol or levels of HDL or LDL cholesterol. Other research reports that having high oxidized LDL levels increases the risk of a heart attack by 400 percent.

Personally, I believe that physicians and the medical industry continue focusing on cholesterol as the cause of heart disease mostly because they have drugs to lower it. The fact is, there's a great deal of money at stake to continue to support and defend this cholesterol hypothesis with almost $18 billion spent annually on statin drugs. We only have a few approved antioxidant drugs, and they're rarely used due to negative side effects.

Another problem that arises when profit-driven drug companies fund the majority of medical research is evident in what statins drugs do to CoQ10 levels. Most practicing and prescribing physicians (as well as drug companies) know that statin drugs negatively affect CoQ10 levels and why this contributes to a statin drug's side effects. Drug companies cannot patent CoQ10 to turn into a drug, so a prescription drug will never be available. Since there are no CoQ10 drugs for a doctor to prescribe, most simply just ignore the problem.

Most conventionally trained medical doctors rarely recommend dietary supplements to their patients even when something like a simple CoQ10 dietary supplement could prevent many of the side effects their patients experience when taking statin drugs. Along the same vein, there are lots of effective natural antioxidant supplements like hibiscus flowers that will never be turned into drugs, and your doctor probably won't be telling you about them or their potential benefits in treating the real underlying cause of clogged arteries. The fact is, conventional doctors are trained and licensed to prescribe drugs—they haven't been trained to prescribe or recommend dietary supplements, and most are just too busy to keep up with the research on dietary supplements to make informed recommendations.

Hibiscus Flower's Ability to Lower Cholesterol

In developing countries where the general population can't afford expensive statin drugs, hibiscus flower tea is used effectively to lower cholesterol levels. This traditional use has also been well studied and scientifically validated through human and animal studies, including double and triple randomized human clinical trials around the world.

Hibiscus flowers were first reported to be able to lower cholesterol in animals in 1991, and 23 different studies have confirmed this action, including nine human studies. Research reports that hibiscus flowers lower total serum cholesterol, low-density lipoprotein (LDL) cholesterol, and serum triglycerides, but high-density lipoprotein cholesterol (HDL—the "good" cholesterol) levels were increased slightly in most clinical studies. Most of the human studies on cholesterol indicate that hibiscus flowers can lower LDL cholesterol by around 7 to 15 points, and it lowers triglycerides levels up to 20 points when using dried hibiscus flowers in a capsule, tablet, or tea bag. Even low dosages of just a single 500-mg tablet taken once daily was reported in 2017 to lower total cholesterol from 196 to 189, LDL decreased from 117 to 107, and HDL was increased from 51 to 56 in one month.

Other researchers used standardized extracts of the flowers that focused on extracting just anthocyanins (and may have left other synergistic beneficial chemicals behind) and reported that cholesterol was lowered but in smaller amounts (5 to 7 points) than was seen with the natural flower tea. While the amount of cholesterol lowered by hibiscus flowers is less than statin drugs (which can lower cholesterol by up to 50 points), statin drugs do not address oxidized cholesterol and inflammation the way hibiscus flowers can.

More doctors and researchers are starting to reevaluate the cholesterol hypothesis; however, there is simply not enough truly unbiased research yet, especially long-term studies, to effectively change the current status quo of recommending very low cholesterol levels. It will be up to you to decide, do your own research, ask your doctor questions, and make informed decisions about your health. And one really good decision is: If you are taking a statin drug and you choose to continue to do so, take a really good CoQ10 supplement regularly. It can make a real difference in reducing negative side effects of the drug and may well reduce your risk of heart failure in the future.

Blood Pressure–Lowering Actions

Another long traditional use of hibiscus flowers in Mexico and Africa is using the tea to treat high blood pressure. While Mexicans have about the same rate of high blood pressure in their population as Americans do, many people in Mexico use a daily hibiscus flower tea instead of the many expensive antihypertensive drugs Americans use to regulate their blood pressure. This traditional use has been well studied and validated in humans and animals with research reporting that hibiscus flowers work quite well for mild to moderate hypertension.

The blood pressure–lowering effect of hibiscus flowers was first recorded by researchers in the African country Senegal in 1962. In the ensuing years, more than 30 different human and animal studies published around the world confirm that hibiscus flowers lower blood pressure effectively. These include 16 human studies, including randomized human clinical trials, which are generally considered the gold standard for all types of medical research.

The leaves and the flower calyces of roselle were studied, and the flower calyces provided much better actions to lower blood pressure than the leaves. Researchers reported that hibiscus flower tea was more effective than the commonly prescribed antihypertensive heart drug captopril and equal to the ACE-inhibitor heart drug lisinopril. One of these studies, published in 2004 by researchers in Mexico, was a randomized controlled human clinical trial. One half of the hypertensive patients took 25 milligrams of captopril twice daily, and the other half took 10 grams of dried hibiscus flowers prepared into a tea once daily. The study revealed that the flower tea was slightly more effective than the antihypertensive drug. At the end of four weeks, the hibiscus flower tea reduced the average blood pressure of patients from 139/91 to 123/79.

In 2010, researchers in the United States confirmed these actions in a randomized, double-blind, placebo-controlled clinical trial with 65 prehypertensive and mildly hypertensive adults. Patients were given 3.75 grams of dried hibiscus flowers brewed into a tea once daily for six weeks. Interestingly, they noted that the hibiscus flower tea was more effective at lowering blood pressure in patients with higher blood pressure levels than those whose levels were only slightly elevated.

In other human studies, systolic blood pressure (SBP) and diastolic blood pressure (DBP) were decreased by 15 and 4 points respectively following daily consumption of 4 grams of hibiscus flowers brewed into a tea for 30 days by patients with type 2 diabetes and mild hypertension. Furthermore, patients with moderate essential hypertension had SBP and DBP decreases of 18 and 11 points respectively following daily consumption of 2 teaspoons of powdered hibiscus flowers in a glass of water for four weeks. In 2014, researchers in Spain gave patients with metabolic syndrome (a feature of which is elevated blood pressure levels) a hibiscus flower extract. They also reported significant drops in blood pressure and reported: "Our primary and most consistent finding is that the consumption of polyphenol-rich HS [hibiscus flower] by humans with metabolic syndrome decreased daytime BP and heart rate, reduced lipid disturbances, and improved oxidative and inflammatory stresses."

The most recent human research on hibiscus flower's ability to treat high blood pressure was published in 2020, and for the first time, it studied the flower's ability to treat high or uncontrolled blood pressure, even while patients were taking prescription drugs to lower their pressure and it wasn't low enough. The pilot study included 29 participants, 72 percent of whom were taking antihypertensive medication due to uncontrolled hypertension and 28 percent of whom were not. At the end of three weeks, 38 percent of the participants reached their target blood pressure and 65 percent saw their systolic blood pressure decrease by at least 10 points. The tea was well tolerated and no side effects were reported, even with those taking prescription blood pressure drugs in combination with the tea.

Animal studies report that hibiscus flowers have vasorelaxant, diuretic, and angiotensin converting enzyme (ACE) inhibitor activities, which are thought to be the main methods in how hibiscus flowers can lower blood pressure. ACE-inhibitor drugs are often prescribed by doctors to treat high blood pressure.

Additionally, four different research studies report on hibiscus flower's diuretic actions, which is thought to contribute to its ability to help lower blood pressure. People with hypertension are often prescribed diuretics to help reduce high blood pressure and fluid retention. The flower tea's diuretic action, when given to hypertensive patients in two studies, were compared to a group of diuretic pharmaceuticals and found to be equally effective. They also reported that the hibiscus treatment did not have any significant effect on electrolytes (which can be a negative side effect of some diuretic drugs).

According to most studies, the overall blood

pressure–lowering effect of hibiscus flowers is related to the flower's ACE-inhibitor actions and a reduction in serum sodium levels through its diuretic actions. Nevertheless, some researchers report that these mechanisms contribute to a lesser degree and that the antioxidant, anti-inflammatory, and endothelium-dependent effects are, most likely, the main mechanisms involved in the blood pressure–lowering effect of hibiscus flowers.

The endothelium is a thin membrane that lines the inside of the heart and blood vessels. Endothelial cells release substances that control the vascular relaxation and constriction of the blood vessels. Endothelial dysfunction has been shown to be of significance in predicting stroke and heart attacks due to the inability of the arteries to dilate fully. When arteries are constricted, blood pressure rises. Chronic inflammation and oxidative stress in endothelial cells are leading causes of endothelial dysfunction. In addition, if endothelial dysfunction remains unaddressed, it can develop into other types of cardiovascular diseases. While hibiscus flower's ability to effectively address inflammation and oxidative stress is highly beneficial to help lower blood pressure by addressing endothelial dysfunction, new research on hibiscus flowers suggests that the flowers can also modulate various substances produced in endothelium cells to promote vasodilation, which, in turn, promotes lower blood pressure. Vasodilator drugs are yet another class of prescription drugs often prescribed for people with high blood pressure.

While scientists continue to argue about which of these effects and mechanisms of actions are playing the most important roles, hibiscus flowers remain an important and effective natural remedy to help lower blood pressure, no matter how the remedy is working. That hibiscus flowers come with other positive benefits as discussed in this book rather than the negative effects of standard prescription drugs used to lower blood pressure makes a good situation even better! With the efficacy and safety of hibiscus flowers for hypertension now confirmed through human studies, it should become a much more popular natural remedy for high blood pressure in the future.

Heart-Protective and Preventative Actions

In addition to the previously discussed cellular-protective antioxidant studies showing that hibiscus flowers can prevent oxidative stress to the heart, other research has reported on beneficial actions to prevent heart damage and cardiovascular diseases. In 2019, researchers in the United Kingdom reported that drinking hibiscus flower tea was beneficial in lowering the risk of cardiovascular diseases (CVD) in a randomized, controlled, single-blind human study. They summarized their study saying that hibiscus flower tea (7.5 grams of dried flowers prepared into a tea and drunk once daily): "improved postprandial vascular function and may be a useful dietary strategy to reduce endothelial dysfunction and CVD risk." They attributed these benefits mainly to the antioxidant and anti-inflammatory benefits of the flower to prevent and repair endothelial dysfunction.

Two different research groups at a medical university in Malaysia published studies in 2019 on the effect of a hibiscus flower tea in rats with induced heart attacks (myocardial infarction). The first group reported that the flower tea effectively treated rats with cardiac hypertrophy (enlargement and thickening of the heart) following a heart attack as well as improved oxidative stress and resulting inflammation to the heart, which is a well-established side effect of having a heart attack. The second group studied the effect for an additional period of time and reported that the flower tea prevented or repaired other deregulations and heart remodeling that occurs after a heart attack and suggested that it could be used as an early adjunctive treatment to prevent future heart failure. One of these groups published a rat study a year earlier that reported these same results, but in a diabetic animal model. The flower tea prevented the cardiovascular remodeling and heart enlargement caused by diabetes in rats and also improved the ability of the heart muscles to contract and relax.

In addition, Nigerian researchers conducted a small study with 25 men who were given a hibiscus flower tea (2.5 grams in 240 milliliters of water) once daily for 30 days. These researchers reported in 2019 that the patients achieved significant improvement in cardiovascular health through various indicators, and they suggested that the tea might prevent cardiovascular disease. In 2015, other researchers in Spain drew the same conclusions when they gave patients hibiscus flower tea.

SUMMARY

Roselle is nature's gift for a healthy heart due to the flower's ability to lower blood pressure and cholesterol levels, prevent and treat clogged arteries, protect the heart, and ward off some of the most common heart diseases. As a natural health practitioner, I have always sought to find and treat the root causes of illness and disease to help my clients rather than just focus on their symptoms. I will continue to recommend hibiscus flowers for heart problems like high blood pressure and cholesterol levels, clogged arteries, and other heart issues because I believe, based on all the research, it truly is addressing many of the root causes of these heart issues. It should be one of the first herbal remedies you turn to if you're experiencing problems with your heart, or better yet, to avoid heart problems. With quality science, including human studies validating these uses, it should be much more popular in the United States than it is today. The main purpose of this book is to help educate people about this heart-healthy natural remedy so it is no longer a secret. I hope you will help share this secret with your friends and family as well. The number of people taking statin and blood pressure drugs is staggering, and the rates of cardiovascular diseases and heart failure are on the rise. Having vital information about healthy and natural alternatives is critical if we, as a society, want to lower our healthcare costs while improving our health.

With hibiscus flower's powerful antioxidant and anti-inflammatory actions, it's not surprising that it has been the subject of other research on diseases and conditions where inflammation and oxidative stress are playing major roles. We'll take a look at this in the next chapter.

CHAPTER 3

More Benefits and Uses of Hibiscus Flowers

With hibiscus flower's powerful antioxidant and anti-inflammatory actions, it's not surprising that it has been the subject of other research on diseases and conditions where inflammation and oxidative stress are playing major roles. This chapter reviews the science and research conducted on this important natural remedy for diabetes, metabolic syndrome, obesity, healthy aging, and more. More than 10,000 studies have been published in the last five years on the negative effects that chronic inflammation and oxidative stress create in our bodies that are now linked as direct causes or contributing factors to many types of diseases and conditions, including Alzheimer's disease, kidney disease, diabetes and other common metabolic diseases, and even just aging.

Anti-Aging and AGE-Inhibitor Actions

These effects bring us to roselle's next researched benefit and action—hibiscus flowers can promote healthy aging. Aging has been associated with a chronic low-grade inflammatory state as well as increased oxidative stress. It is widely accepted that reactive oxygen species (ROS) in many cells accumulates over our lifespan and leads to a state of chronic oxidative stress at old age. Low-grade inflammation caused by oxidative stress is also now strongly linked to much higher risks of developing age-related memory loss, dementia, and even Alzheimer's disease. Hibiscus flower's ability to effectively reduce chronic inflammation and oxidative stress will help promote healthy aging. Several studies on hibiscus flowers report these actions.

One of the most recent studies on hibiscus flower's anti-aging action was an industry-standard test. Researchers have developed a special mutated species of flat worm (*Caenorhabditis elegans*) that they regularly use for anti-aging research. If a plant or a substance can prolong the short lifespan of this particular worm, it indicates that the substance might also help prolong the life of humans. Usually plants and plant chemicals passing this test are targeted for further anti-aging research to determine their specific actions in this regard.

Researchers in Germany published a study in 2019 reporting that a hibiscus flower extract increased the lifespan of this special worm by 24 percent and noted it was more than the just one chemical they tested (hydroxycitric acid) that provided these results. Their study also reported that the hibiscus extract elicited a strong protection against amyloid-ß-induced toxicity. This is the small protein linked to brain cell death and the progression of Alzheimer's disease.

Researchers in Switzerland reported that the polysaccharides in hibiscus flower may provide anti-aging benefits to the skin. Their *in vitro* study published in 2004 revealed that these natural compounds could increase the production of and increase the differentiation of skin cells called keratinocytes, which can strengthen aging skin that has become thin and fragile. More recently, a research group in Taiwan and another in Singapore both published studies in 2019 indicating that hibiscus flower tea provided anti-aging benefits to the skin. They reported that a water extract of hibiscus flowers was a natural antioxidant with the ability to maintain collagen production, to decrease melanin syntheses under UVB radiation, reduce ROS created by sun exposure, and to increase mitochondrial function in skin cells.

Another huge area of anti-aging research over the last 10 years indicates that reducing advanced glycation end products (AGEs) in the body provides anti-aging benefits. AGEs are harmful compounds that are formed when protein or fat combines or bonds improperly with sugar in the bloodstream. This process is called glycation. These improperly bonded compounds can travel throughout the body and cause a host of problems, including chronic inflammation, cellular damage and cell death, and the interruption of cellular signaling. AGEs also encourage the creation of ROS, which generate oxidative stress and more inflammation. In fact, AGEs and ROS are uniquely intertwined. For an AGE to be created inside the body, the protein or the fat that creates the bond has to be oxidized first, usually by ROS. Therefore, having higher ROS levels means having more AGEs. Once an AGE is created, the damage and inflammation it causes results in the formation of more ROS, and a negative cycle is established.

AGEs and the damage they cause are now linked to cellular aging and premature aging inside the body and in various organs. Over a dozen different AGEs have been identified in the human body and about half are known to accumulate with age in skin cells, affecting collagen production and promoting wrinkling and thinning of the skin. The rest of the AGEs can start accumulating in other organs and in the bloodstream, causing aging and cellular damage in the heart, kidneys, liver, and brain, resulting in chronic age-related diseases in these organs.

The link between AGEs and age-related diseases was recognized as early as 2001, when medical researchers at the University of South Carolina reported in the journal *Experimental Gerontology* that "they [AGEs] accumulate to high levels in tissues in age-related chronic diseases, such as atherosclerosis, diabetes, arthritis and neurodegenerative disease. Inhibition of AGE formation in these diseases may limit oxidative and inflammatory damage in tissues, retarding the progression of pathophysiology and improve the quality of life during aging." Recently, measuring AGE levels in individuals over age 60 has been proposed as a possible new blood test to monitor healthy aging and to enable the early detection of age-related diseases.

Hibiscus Flower's AGE-Inhibitor Actions

Researchers in Taiwan reported in 2011 that a hibiscus polyphenol extract (HPE) had a direct action against AGEs. Their study used a type 2 diabetic rat model since animals and humans with diabetes produce a significant amount of AGEs and suffer from well-known AGE-damage to various organs. These researchers summarized their research thusly: "Diabetes promoted plasma advanced glycation end product (AGE) formation and lipid peroxidation [oxidation of fats], while HPE significantly reduced these elevations." They also noted that the hibiscus extract also disabled the receptor sites for AGEs in the heart, so the AGEs didn't migrate to those receptor sites to cause cellular damage in that organ. At least seven natural compounds in hibiscus flowers have been individually tested and confirmed with AGE-inhibitor actions, which are thought to be delivering these important benefits.

The confirmed actions of hibiscus flower's ability to reduce ROS, AGEs, oxidative stress, and chronic inflammation can promote healthy aging in numerous ways. Natural plant antioxidants, including those found in hibiscus flowers, have long been documented to prevent many age-related diseases, including heart disease, diabetes, cancer, neurodegenerative diseases, osteoporosis, and many others. In fact, researchers in Spain reported in 2018 that hibiscus flowers could be beneficial in the treatment or prevention of age-related macular degeneration and released an earlier preliminary report in 2017 (based on test-tube studies) indicating that the flowers may also be beneficial for age-related osteoporosis.

Antidiabetic Actions

All the previously discussed AGE-inhibitor and cellular-protective antioxidant abilities of hibiscus flower holds important information for people with diabetes. Diabetes causes a significant amount of additional ROS and AGEs in numerous ways, which results in a chronic state of inflammation and oxidative stress.

It is well documented in thousands of studies that oxidative stress, chronic inflammation, and the resulting cellular damage caused by ROS and AGEs are a significant cause or cofactor of most diabetic complications, such as cardiovascular diseases, kidney damage resulting in renal failure, liver damage and fatty liver, nerve damage resulting in diabetic neuropathy, and macular degeneration. For these reasons, everyone with diabetes should consider eating an antioxidant-rich diet (lots of fresh vegetables and fruits) and taking strong cellular-protective antioxidant herbal remedies like hibiscus flowers if they want to avoid diabetic complications and co-occurring diseases.

Cellular-protective antioxidants and AGE inhibitors like those found in hibiscus flowers may allow people with diabetes to live longer and manage their diabetes much more easily by avoiding many of these debilitating diabetic complications by effectively reducing ROS and

AGEs, and the chronic inflammation and oxidative stress they cause. For more information on why antioxidants in general are very beneficial for diabetes, see my blog article: "What Every Diabetic Needs to Know About Antioxidants" on www.rain-tree.com.

Much of the animal research documenting hibiscus flower's cellular-protective antioxidant actions previously discussed to protect the heart, kidneys, brain, and liver were performed on diabetic animals. In addition, a 2018 study reported that a hibiscus flower tea was effective for diabetes-associated cognitive impairment. (See the reference section for a list these studies.)

In addition to helping avoid diabetic complications, hibiscus flowers have been documented with direct antidiabetic actions in several other animal studies, mostly by improving insulin sensitivity and/or reducing blood sugar levels. Researchers in Nigeria reported in 2019 that blood sugar levels were reduced in diabetic rats and attributed this action to the flower's ability to reduce absorption of dietary sugars and starches by inhibiting digestive enzymes that are required for their breakdown and absorption. They reported that gallic acid and protocatechuic acid are the natural compounds in hibiscus flower that inhibited these enzymes. (More information on the enzyme-inhibitor actions of hibiscus flowers is found in the upcoming section on weight loss.)

Researchers in Taiwan reported in 2014 that hibiscus flower's antidiabetic actions were attributed to the flower's ability to improve insulin resistance in the liver. In fact, they compared hibiscus flowers with the antidiabetic drug linagliptin, which is used for this purpose, and reported the flower's actions equaled that of the drug in their animal study. Another research group in Thailand studied the use of hibiscus flowers in healthy and diabetic rats and reported an antidiabetic effect of the flowers in 2013. However, they reported a different mechanism of action: Their study reported that administering the animals a hibiscus extract lowered blood glucose levels significantly (by 38 percent) in diabetic rats, but the nondiabetic rats had no change in blood glucose levels.

These researchers also reported that the extract significantly increased the amount of insulin the pancreas produced, and this stimulatory action was twice as strong in diabetic rats over nondiabetic rats. Interestingly, the researchers also noted all hibiscus-treated animals (both diabetic and nondiabetic) significantly increased the number of islets of Langerhans (groups of specialized cells in the pancreas that make and secrete hormones, including insulin). An increase in the number of these cells may help explain the higher insulin levels noted in the animals. These special cells are often the target of cellular damage by AGEs and ROS, which can reduce insulin secretion in diabetics.

Newer research published in 2019 confirmed these actions when researchers reported that hibiscus flowers were able to help regenerate and/or repair pancreatic beta cells in the islets of Langerhans in a type 1 diabetes animal model. Other researchers in Indonesia noticed some these same effects when they administered hibiscus flowers to diabetic rats; however, they reported yet another mechanism of action in their research: They reported that the flowers had a direct effect on a hormone called glucagon-like peptide 1 (GLP-1). GLP-1 plays a role in the pancreas to increase insulin secretion, stimulate proliferation (cell growth), and prevent pancreatic beta cell death (apoptosis). This hormone is much lower in diabetics, and the hibiscus flower treatment was reported to return GLP-1 to normal levels in diabetic rats.

Scientists are just beginning to understand how specifically hibiscus flowers might positively affect diabetes. With all these benefits working in many different ways, it's of little wonder that hibiscus flower tea has long been recommended to people with diabetes by herbal healers and alternative health practitioners throughout Mexico.

If you are diabetic, check with your doctor before using hibiscus flowers—as you should before taking any herbal supplements. Your blood sugar levels should be closely monitored and tested more frequently until you determine how hibiscus flowers affect your glucose levels. If you experience even some of the benefits outlined here, you'll need your doctor's help to determine if your prescribed diabetic medications need adjusting. As some of these mechanisms of action work slowly with an accumulative effect, continue testing regularly as long as you are taking this natural remedy.

Weight-Loss Actions

The most recent area of research on hibiscus flowers may well be the most exciting one after its positive effects for our hearts. Twenty-five human and animal studies report that hibiscus flowers can help us lose weight. The first way hibiscus flowers promote weight loss is by lowering the calories in the foods we eat. Natural compounds in the flowers interfere with the three main digestive enzymes that break down fats, starches, and sugars. These enzymes (pancreatic lipase, alpha-amylase, and alpha-glucosidase) are responsible for breaking down food into small enough molecules so that they can be absorbed in the stomach and intestines. If these enzymes don't do their job, these larger fat, sugar, and starch molecules (and their calories) aren't absorbed and are just eliminated through the stools. This makes whatever is eaten lower in calories. These enzyme-inhibiting actions with regard to sugar and starch absorption have also been linked to how hibiscus flowers are able to lower blood sugar levels in the diabetic research previously discussed.

The second way hibiscus flowers promote weight loss is by interfering with adipogenesis, the natural process the body uses to create new fat cells. When this process is reduced, fewer fat cells are created, and less fat is stored in fatty tissues.

Another method that promotes weight loss is through the flower's well-documented antioxidant and anti-inflammatory actions. New research on obesity indicates that obesity is actually a chronic inflammatory disease, and the fatty tissues of overweight individuals are inflamed and suffering from oxidative stress. When fat cells and fatty tissues are damaged by inflammation and oxidative stress, they do not produce enough of certain natural metabolic chemicals that are required to reduce inflammation, store and burn fats, maintain insulin sensitivity, and support a healthy weight. This can make losing weight much harder and even promotes weight gain. For more information on why antioxidant and anti-inflammatory agents are the newest method to achieve weight loss and/or treat obesity (which also makes maintaining a healthier weight much easier), see my blog article "Why Antioxidants Help You Lose Weight" on www.rain-tree.com.

The last way hibiscus flowers encourage weight loss is through the flower's actions on the gut microbiome. All the species of bacteria and other small microbes that reside in our gut is what makes up the gut microbiome, with the largest number residing in the colon. Ten years of research around the world on the gut microbiome reveals that the number and types of bacteria in our gut play an important role in regulating our weight. In fact, the gut microbiome is now considered an important "metabolic organ" in our bodies for this reason. Within all this research, natural polyphenols, like those found in hibiscus flowers, have emerged as effective natural agents that are capable of killing off particular bacterial species that are elevated, while encouraging the growth of other beneficial species that are diminished in overweight people, in a manner that modulates the overall gut microbiome to encourage weight loss.

I spent more than a year researching the ability of plant polyphenols and flavonoids to promote weight loss through these four mechanisms while I was writing a book on a rainforest fern. Interestingly, both plants are great sources of natural chemicals with antioxidant, anti-inflammatory, bacteria-modulating, and enzyme-inhibitor actions. During this research, I tested overweight people taking both plants and read thousands of studies on these important plant chemicals and how they promote weight loss. The end result of my personal research revealed that the synergy of all these natural polyphenols and flavonoids working together is the key to the benefits these plants provide for weight loss.

I also discovered that the combination of chemicals in the fern worked much better for weight loss while the combination of active polyphenols in hibiscus flowers worked much better for high cholesterol, high blood pressure, and clogged arteries. For example, while hibiscus flowers have five natural chemicals known to be enzyme inhibitors, which can lower the calories in food, the fern contains 21 known enzyme inhibitors, some of which were reported to work more effectively at much lower dosages. Simultaneously, hibiscus flowers contain certain polyphenols that are known to lower blood pressure that are not present in the fern.

For these reasons, I believe that people taking hibiscus flowers for their heart health may notice a beneficial "side effect" of losing a little weight and those taking the fern for weight loss may notice a beneficial side effect of a little better heart function. For more information on how plant enzyme inhibitors, anti-inflammatories, antioxidants, and bacteria-modulating actions can help promote weight loss, visit my Author Page on Amazon.com for updates on other books in this series and specifically *Nature's Secret for Weight Loss*. Nevertheless, hibiscus flowers have been the subject of research that report the flowers can indeed promote weight loss, as discussed next.

The Studies on Weight-Loss Actions

At least a dozen animal studies, several *in vitro* (test tube) studies, and one human study to date report hibiscus flower's weight-loss actions. While some researchers reported polyphenols or anthocyanins as the main active chemicals providing these actions, other authors concluded in their research that other organic acids and their derivatives (hibiscus acids and hydroxycitric acids) contained in the flowers were responsible for the beneficial effects observed in their studies. As is often the case with medicinal plants, the effects were probably achieved through the synergistic action of many chemicals they tested working together.

The published research supports the mechanisms of actions described earlier—inhibiting digestive enzymes and the formation of fat cells, relieving oxidative stress and chronic inflammation, and modulating the gut microbiome. (See References for a listing of these studies.)

The human weight-loss study was conducted by a research group at the Institute of Medicine, Chung Shan Medical University in Taiwan and published in 2014. It was a double-blind placebo-controlled trial with 40 obese subjects. Half of the subjects were given a freeze-dried hibiscus flower water extract in capsules (taken after each meal), and half were given a placebo (starch pills). The results they noted in this human study were not as dramatic as were observed in the previous animal studies on the unextracted flowers. At the end of 12 weeks of supplementing with hibiscus flowers, 70 percent of the study subjects taking the flowers lost weight, and those losing weight lost an average of about three pounds at the end of 12 weeks. In addition, weight circumference in all subjects taking hibiscus flowers was reduced by almost an inch, and body fat percentage fell from 37.37 to 36.67. While the researchers noted that these results were a "significant reduction" compared to the placebo group, I don't think the overall weight loss achieved over 12 weeks to be all that significant.

As I indicated earlier, I will still continue to recommend the weight-loss fern I studied over hibiscus flowers for weight loss, and tell people they might notice an additional benefit of losing a little weight (especially belly weight, it seems) when they take hibiscus flowers as a heart remedy. It just works much better for the heart (and much better than the fern works for the heart) than it does for weight loss.

Metabolic Syndrome Management

With hibiscus flower's ability to reduce belly fat, increase insulin sensitivity, reduce blood pressure and cholesterol levels, and protect the heart, it is of little wonder that hibiscus flowers are being studied as a new herbal remedy for metabolic syndrome.

Metabolic syndrome (MetS) is defined by a clustering of metabolic disorders that include increased belly fat and weight gain, deregulated cholesterol levels, insulin resistance and deregulated blood sugar levels, and nonoptimal blood pressure levels. Depending on how cholesterol and fat metabolism is deregulated, nonalcoholic fatty liver disease can also be one of the metabolic disorders in MetS. MetS is associated with a much greater risk of developing cardiovascular diseases and type 2 diabetes. The Centers for Disease Control (CDC) reports the prevalence of MetS is estimated at more than 30 percent of the population in the United States today.

If you have MetS, here's an important bit of "insider" information you need: When scientists go into the laboratory to study MetS in animals to see if certain drugs or natural remedies like hibiscus flowers can treat the condition, they must first induce MetS in the animals to be able to conduct their studies. Researchers have an easy way to give animals MetS—they just feed the animals a high-fructose diet for six to eight weeks. That means lowering or eliminating excess fructose (especially the high-fructose corn syrup found in sodas and other processed foods) in your diet is certainly helpful and highly recommended if you suffer from this metabolic disorder. When your body processes high-fructose sugars, significant numbers of ROS and AGEs are created, and high-fructose diets have been reported to reduce the amount and/or the actions of the natural antioxidants that the body usually produces to keep ROS and AGEs in check. Most of the research reports that oxidative stress and inflammation are involved in the association between obesity, insulin resistance, and hypertension and note that antioxidant and anti-inflammatory plant components like polyphenols might be useful as a treatment for MetS.

Five recent animal studies and one human study report that a hibiscus flower tea may well be a highly effective herbal remedy for this common metabolic condition. The animal studies confirmed hibiscus flower's ability to lower blood pressure, cholesterol, triglycerides, and blood sugar levels, as well as relieve oxidative stress. Most of these researchers concluded that hibiscus flowers should be further studied as a natural remedy for MetS.

The human study was published in 2010 by researchers in Mexico where the prevalence of MetS is even higher than in the United States. Eighty healthy volunteers were recruited to form a control group and compared to 72 patients with MetS. All subjects were given an extract of hibiscus flowers in a dosage of only 100 milligrams once daily. The MetS patients taking the flower extract demonstrated significant improvements in all of the parameters tested—cholesterol and triglycerides, blood pressure, insulin sensitivity, and blood glucose levels. The researchers reported that hibiscus flowers could be considered beneficial in the clinical management of MetS.

Infection-Fighting Actions

Another large body of research pertains to hibiscus flower's ability to kill bacteria, viruses, and fungi. A flower tea has been used as an herbal remedy in many countries for various types of internal and external bacterial infections, as well as some viral and fungal infections. Recent research has now validated some of these uses.

Twenty-nine studies published between 2008 and 2019 confirm that hibiscus flowers can kill many types of bacteria, viruses, and fungi. In fact, extracts of the flowers now have the FDA's and the European Union's equivalent of "generally regarded as safe" (GRAS) food status as a food additive to reduce or eliminate some food-spoilage microorganisms and foodborne bacteria that cause illness. Its approval as a food additive is also for the purpose of a natural flavoring ingredient and a natural red food coloring for food and beverages. (See the reference section for a listing of these studies.)

One human study reported that a hibiscus flower tea was highly effective in treating recurring urinary tract infections (bacterial and candida) in pregnant women without toxicity or side effects. The flower tea has also been reported to kill various species of bacteria found in the mouth that cause dental plaque, cavities, and periodontal diseases. These antibacterial actions against mouth bacteria is important information for those taking hibiscus flowers for heart conditions.

Interestingly, mouth bacteria that causes periodontal disease over time may increase the risk of clogged arteries, heart disease, and stroke. Many studies have shown that people with periodontal disease may be two to three times more likely to have coronary artery disease than people with healthy mouths. Periodontal disease is a chronic inflammatory disease that slowly and steadily destroys the supporting structures of multiple teeth.

Scientists have proposed several possible explanations for the association between heart disease and periodontal disease. One is that the bacteria that causes periodontal disease release inflammatory toxins into the bloodstream, which can contribute to arterial plaque by recruiting immune cells to deal with the bacterial toxins, which increases the formation of foam cells that contribute to arterial plaque. Another explanation is that these bacteria and their toxins cause the liver to make high levels of certain proteins, which inflame the blood vessels. Additionally, it is long thought that oral bacteria (typically streptococci bacteria) invades the blood circulation through small ulcers in gum tissue. The bacteria cause platelets in the circulatory system to build up and create blood clots, which can cause heart attacks and strokes. Unfortunately, these same mouth bacteria have also been found in the lining of the heart, causing an infection called endocarditis as well as in the brain of patients who have had strokes.

If you are drinking hibiscus tea for your heart, swish it around in your mouth first before swallowing to keep your gums and teeth healthy, reduce chronic gum inflammation, and address the mouth bacteria that puts you at higher risk to harm your heart. It's also a great natural remedy just for periodontal disease and to reduce bacterial plaque in your mouth.

Cancer-Preventative and Anticancer Actions

Hibiscus flower's cancer preventative and anticancer actions have been documented in 15 test-tube studies and one animal study. All the anticancer research is quite preliminary and are *in vitro* studies—introducing hibiscus flowers to various cancer cells in test tubes to determine which types of cancer cells are killed and how. The preliminary research reveals that the types of cancer cells most susceptible to the actions of the flowers in these studies include gastric cancers, melanoma, leukemia, and multiple myeloma. However, how hibiscus flowers interact with cancer cells inside a test tube can be quite different from how it might react with cancer cells inside the human body. There are no animal or human studies indicating that hibiscus flowers can treat cancer, and as such, hibiscus flowers are not recommended as a natural remedy for cancer.

Thousands of studies however confirm the general cancer-preventative abilities of plant antioxidants, including many of the flower's powerful polyphenols and flavonoids, which are strong antioxidants. Personally, I just view that information as a possible "healthy side effect" when I recommend the flowers for other conditions for which hibiscus flowers are quite effective.

One animal study suggests that hibiscus flowers might provide cancer-preventative actions. When researchers administered a flower tea to animals, it prevented healthy cells from mutating into cancerous cells when given a substance known to create mutations. Since most of the strong cellular-protective antioxidant chemicals in hibiscus flowers have been shown to have good antimutagenic actions, it is not very surprising that the flowers evidenced this cancer-preventative action.

Kidney Stone and Gout Prevention

In several countries, hibiscus flowers have been traditionally used for kidney stones and gout. Six studies (including two human studies) report that the flowers may help to prevent the formation of kidney stones, which confirm these traditional uses.

There are basically four different types of stones that are formed by too much of a certain substance that is present in the kidneys, including calcium oxalate, calcium phosphate, uric acid, or cystine. Some of these substances come from the types of food we're eating. The relapse rate for kidney stones is above 50 percent, which means if you've had kidney stones in the past, you're more likely to develop them again.

The juice of hibiscus flowers was first studied for the prevention of kidney stones in humans by researchers in Thailand in 1994. This study reported that after consumption of the flower juice by 36 healthy volunteers, the urine showed a decrease of uric acid, calcium, and phosphate. In 2008, these Thailand university researchers published another study that compared the effect of hibiscus flowers in subjects who had previously had kidney stones to those who had not. The volunteers' urine was analyzed for uric acid and oxalate and other chemical compositions related to kidney stone risk factors. Their results indicated that the flowers were capable of substantially increasing the excretion and clearance of oxalate and uric acid, which would be beneficial for uric acid–type and oxalate-type kidney stones, as well as gout (which is generally caused by high uric acid levels). These results were achieved by giving subjects a cup of tea made from 1.5 grams of dried hibiscus flowers twice daily (morning and evening) for 15 days. Researchers noted that the flower tea lowered the risk of stone formation in both groups, but the prevention benefit was much higher in the group who previously had kidney stones.

These results were confirmed in an animal study published in 2011 by a different university in Thailand. These researchers reported that when rats were given hibiscus flowers, there was a significant decrease in serum oxalate and glycolate, higher oxalate urinary excretion, and decreased calcium crystal deposition in the kidneys.

Other Areas of Study

The sedative and anti-anxiety actions of the flower tea were confirmed in one animal study, and the antispasmodic, antidiarrhea, and wound-healing actions were confirmed in other animal studies. (See the reference section for a listing of these research studies.)

CHAPTER 4

A Consumer Guide
for Hibiscus Flowers

Hibiscus flower remedies have been gaining in popularity around the world for many of the uses discussed in this book. While much of the newest research hasn't been widely circulated in the U.S. natural products market, word is slowly getting out. Hibiscus flower tea bags have been around for a couple of years and in 2019 several new hibiscus flower herbal supplements in capsules became available in the United States. Prior to that, consumers' only options were to purchase hibiscus flowers in bulk and prepare their own tea with them. With hibiscus flowers providing the first real alternatives to statin drugs and for treating mild to moderate high blood pressure for millions of Americans, the market for this interesting, pretty, and powerful heart-healthy flower should grow quickly.

Traditional Preparation

The traditional remedy is to prepare a standard decoction with the dried flowers. Take one ounce (about 30 grams) of chopped dried hibiscus flowers and boil gently in 4 cups of water for 10 minutes. Remove from the heat and allow to steep for 10 minutes and then strain the flowers out of the decoction. Manufactured tea bags can be used by the cup or the liter instead if desired: determine the number of tea bags necessary based on how many grams of flowers the tea bags contain, which can vary. To prepare it by the cup, use 2 tablespoons cut-up dried flowers or 2 teaspoons of flowers ground into a powder.

This decoction is quite sour and is usually sweetened to taste with sugar, honey, or stevia. In traditional herbal medicine systems, 1 cup of the decoction is drunk once or twice daily with the remaining refrigerated. Also, don't forget to swish the tea around in your mouth before swallowing for healthier teeth and gums!

The Safety of Hibiscus Flowers

The very long history of use of hibiscus flowers as a food and a medicine throughout the world has established that this natural remedy is well tolerated with few, if any, side effects. The many human studies conducted on the flowers over the years have also noted no toxic effects. Hibiscus flower has even been studied in pregnant women with no ill effects to mother or baby. The plant has been awarded GRAS-status (generally recognized as safe) by several government agencies as a food additive, which is the final indication that the remedy is generally safe to use.

However, that doesn't mean that hibiscus flowers should not be treated as a medicinal plant with specific biological activities. These actions may have an effect when people are taking prescription drugs. If you have been prescribed a prescription drug, it is always advisable to check with your healthcare provider before taking any herbal remedy, including hibiscus flowers. Herb-drug interaction studies are expensive to conduct and are rarely all-encompassing, so it's best to err on the side of caution. Along those lines, please review the possible contraindications and drug interactions and check with your healthcare provider if you have any concerns.

Contraindications

❏ Do not use hibiscus flowers while breastfeeding. One rat study reported late onset of puberty in juvenile rats whose mothers consumed roselle tea prior to weaning.

❏ Hibiscus flowers are a natural source of iron and have been used to treat anemia in some countries with mixed results. If you have hemochromatosis (high iron levels), you should avoid using this remedy.

Drug Interactions

❏ May potentiate and/or increase the effect of diuretic and antihypertensive drugs. Check your blood pressure regularly to determine the flower's effect on your blood pressure and consult with your doctor if your medications need adjusting.

❑ May potentiate and/or increase the effect of anti-inflammatory drugs. One human study reported that combining the flower tea with a common NSAID anti-inflammatory drug, diclofenac, resulted in less of the drug being excreted in urine, which might cause an additive or increase the effect of the drug. Use with caution or seek the advice of your health practitioner if you are regularly taking anti-inflammatory drugs.

❑ One human study with six healthy subjects reported that hibiscus flowers taken as a single dose with a statin drug sped the clearance of the statin drug from the liver, which led researchers to suggest the flowers might cause a reduced effect of the statin drug. However, this study measured just a single dose. These same researchers administered hibiscus flowers in combination with a statin drug to laboratory animals for 30 days and reported the flowers had an added effect and lowered cholesterol levels greater than the statin drug alone produced. While the flowers might clear the statin from the liver more quickly, hibiscus flower remedies taken with statins regularly may increase the effectiveness of statin drugs.

Finding a Good Hibiscus Flower Product

A growing number of roselle/hibiscus flower herbal products are available in the United States today. Several products are offered in tea bags that have around 5 to 6 grams of cut-up dried hibiscus flowers inside each tea bag. Several companies that offer bulk herb supplies offer dried hibiscus flowers by the ounce and the pound, and these are often the most cost-effective product to purchase. Putting a couple tablespoons of the dried flowers in a pot of water to boil into the herbal remedy isn't difficult, and many will boil enough of the dried flowers to fill a 1- to 2-quart pitcher to keep in the refrigerator for daily use. This is especially true in the hot summer, since a glass of iced hibiscus tea has a beneficial cooling effect and can lower your body temperature.

Bulk supplies of hibiscus flowers are currently shipped into the United States and abroad from Mexico, Brazil, several African countries, China, and Thailand, where major cultivation programs are expanding to meet the growing world demand for hibiscus natural remedies.

Do look for a certified organic source of flowers, regardless of the type of product purchased. Many of these developing nations have different laws and regulations about pesticides that may be allowed in foods and medicinal plants that are banned in the United States. The flower calyces are sweet and juicy and can be preyed on by various insects; therefore, some growers may use insecticides to protect their crops. The most troublesome contaminate, however, is mold and fungi. These plants are growing in the moist and humid tropics, the calyces are moist and juicy, and care must be used in harvesting and drying to avoid mold and fungus.

Natural Flowers versus Flower Extracts

Newer on the market are capsules of the dried flowers, and these include just dried, powdered flowers stuffed into capsules, as well as concentrated 4:1 extracts and standardized extracts sold in capsules. Consumers should always ask questions about these extract products because they can be a bit misleading by being marketed as much stronger than the natural flowers, which supposedly allows lower dosages to be taken.

However, with a medicinal plant like hibiscus, the efficacy of these products really are all about the chemistry of the plant you start with and how many and how much of the natural chemicals were extracted in their manufacturing process and are delivered in the extract. The fact is, hibiscus flowers are rich in organic acids, polyphenols, anthocyanins, fiber, polysaccharides, and volatile constituents that have health benefits. Research has been funded on this natural remedy because all these different chemicals work together synergistically and provide greater actions and benefits together than the single chemicals provide alone.

Most standard 4:1 concentrated extracts employed for medicinal plants uses alcohol and high heat, and some natural chemicals (especially some delicate water-soluble polyphenol antioxidant chemicals) will be degraded or not extracted due to the alcohol and heat in this extraction method. Other extracts of hibiscus flowers are called standardized extracts, which are created to guarantee a certain level of active natural compounds in a supplement. These also typically use alcohol and high heat in their manufacturing process, so not all the beneficial chemicals will necessarily be present in the finished product.

With hibiscus flower extracts, consumers need to evaluate these standardized extracts closely. For example, a hibiscus flower extract is sold in 250-mg capsules that is labeled as "guaranteed to contain 12.5 mg [5%] flavones per capsule." The flavones in the flower are some (but not all) of the chemicals delivering antioxidant actions, including the beneficial anthocyanins hibiscus is well known for. What's more, dried natural unextracted hibiscus flowers were reported in one published study to contain about 148 milligrams of flavones in a gram (or 37 mg in 250 mg). Other studies report the flowers contain about 15 to 20 percent flavones per gram of dried flowers. So, in this example, the hibiscus flower extract is not delivering the same amount of flavones as occur in the natural flowers. Therefore, consumers are paying more for this "concentrated extract" (and told they can take less) while the natural flower delivers over twice as much flavones as the standardized extract does.

You will typically pay more for concentrated and standardized extracts, so make sure you're getting what you're paying for or stick with the natural ground-up hibiscus flowers in capsules or tea bags. Some standardized extracts or polyphenol extracts were used in the clinical studies of the flowers in humans and animals in other countries. However, the potency of these extracts were much higher in the research than those sold in the American natural products market today. Some of these researched standardized extracts contained 250 milligrams of total anthocyanins (a type of flavone) per capsule, not just 12.5 milligrams.

Scientists have studied flavones, polyphenols, and other plant antioxidant chemicals for many years and most note that higher amounts of these important plant compounds are required for therapeutic effects. The current extracts of hibiscus flower should not be taken in lower dosages if they are delivering fewer of these compounds than are found in the natural flower. Personally, I will save my money and go natural.

Where to Purchase Hibiscus Flowers

Hibiscus flower products are sold under various names, including roselle, roselle tea, hibiscus flowers, or simply hibiscus tea. Available products include capsules, tea bags, and bulk flowers either in tea-cut or powder sold by the ounce or pound. All of these products should be using the same scientific name on their labels: *Hibiscus sabdariffa*. Most of the products and brands can be purchased through many online retailers including Amazon. com. Some health food stores and larger grocery stores that sell various boxed organic teas may carry hibiscus tea in tea bags, and some health food stores will have hibiscus flowers in tea bags and in capsules as well.

In the United States, during the summer months,

many Hispanic grocery stores offer bulk one-pound bags of dried hibiscus flowers at very reasonable prices in their produce sections since the flower tea is a popular cooling and delicious beverage in Latin American cultures. However, these may not always be organic, so read the label carefully. In fact, the flavor is so enjoyed in these cultures, instant powdered Kool-Aid–like drink mixes (called "Jamaica") are sold and are very popular in Latin American countries and many Latino food markets here in the United States. Keep in mind, however, these drink mixes mostly use the flowers as a flavoring ingredient and to produce the characteristic red-colored drink—not to provide enough of the flowers to be used as a natural remedy for therapeutic purposes.

SUGGESTED DOSAGES FOR HIBISCUS FLOWERS

The dosages used in traditional medicine systems in Mexico and Africa are generally 30 grams (1 ounce) of dried hibiscus flowers per liter of water (about 4 cups). This equates to about 7.5 grams (about 2 tablespoons) of dried flowers per 8 ounces (1 cup) of water if prepared as a single cup of tea. See "Traditional Preparation" earlier in this chapter, which covers how to prepare a standard decoction with the flowers using traditional methods. Bulk loose tea (dried flowers) can be used as well as the more convenient prefilled tea bags. The number of tea bags needed will depend on how much hibiscus flower is contained inside the tea bags (which can vary by manufacturer) and how much liquid is used.

■ FOR HIGH BLOOD PRESSURE

Drink one (8-ounce) cup of a flower tea one to three times daily using 5 grams of dried flowers per 8 ounces or take 2 to 4 grams in capsules twice daily (based on body weight). Dosages used in the human clinical studies ranged from a single 500-milligram capsule taken once daily up to 10 to 20 grams of flowers prepared into a tea and taken daily. The newest research indicates that higher blood pressure levels require higher dosages of the flowers. Doctors started these hypertensive patients on a tea with 5 grams of flowers daily and increased the dosage by 5 grams each week until targeted blood pressure levels were achieved.

Start with one (8-ounce) cup daily for the first week and increase to two (8-ounce cups) daily the following week if levels still need to be lower. Thereafter, an additional cup of tea daily can be taken or more flowers can be used per cup to reach targeted levels. Make sure to check your blood pressure at least twice daily to determine how the flowers are affecting your blood pressure and contact your doctor if your medications need adjusting.

■ FOR CHOLESTEROL AND CLOGGED ARTERIES

If you are taking hibiscus flowers for blood pressure benefits, you will be taking a dosage high enough to address cholesterol and clogged arteries. The dosages used in the human studies for cholesterol also varied widely, and the effective dosages I've recommended for many years are 2 grams in capsules once or twice daily or one (8-ounce) cup of flower tea with 10 grams of flowers per 8 ounces once or twice daily, depending on body weight. If you weigh more than 180 pounds, take the recommended dosage twice daily instead once daily. Also if you have lifestyle factors that promote added ROS and AGEs (if you're a smoker, overweight, or have diabetes), take the higher dosage.

■ FOR HEALTHY AGING AND ANTIOXIDANT BENEFITS

Drink one (8-ounce) cup of a standard flower decoction daily or take 1 to 3 grams in capsules daily. Again, dosages should be adjusted based on body weight and lifestyle factors that may increase your oxidative stress levels (take more if you're a smoker, have diabetes, are overweight, or have other free radical–producing conditions). Take 1 gram daily if you are normal weight and have regular lifestyle factors; take 2 grams daily if you have increased weight or higher lifestyle factors; and take 3 grams daily if you have higher weight and higher lifestyle factors.

■ FOR WEIGHT LOSS

Take 1 to 2 grams in capsules (depending on the size of the meal) 15 to 20 minutes prior to each meal. Capsules are better than teas as they are digested along with the sugar, starches, and fats in the meals to provide blocking actions when digestive enzymes are released during digestion. The natural flowers are also a source of beneficial fiber with weight-loss benefits and the fiber will be missing in the tea but present in the natural flower capsules. For weight loss, it is best to avoid vegetable-based capsules (called veggi caps) and stick with plain gelatin capsules. Veggi caps are slow to dissolve, often not releasing their contents until they're in the intestines. For weight loss purposes, you want the flowers released quickly in the stomach where they're digested along with foods to start blocking digestive enzymes immediately.

■ FOR DIABETES

Drink one (8-ounce) cup of a standard flower decoction twice daily or take 2 to 3 grams (depending on body weight) in capsules twice daily. Make sure to check your blood sugar levels at least twice daily and contact your doctor if your medications need adjusting.

■ FOR COLDS, FLU, UPPER RESPIRATORY INFECTIONS, AND SORE THROATS

Drink one (8-ounce) cup of a warm standard flower decoction twice daily.

Conclusion

According to the latest statistics by American Heart Association, 48 percent of all adults in the United States have some type of cardiovascular disease, largely driven by the high number of people with high blood pressure. Cardiovascular disease (CVD) remains the number-one killer of all Americans, claiming almost 850,000 lives annually. With hibiscus flowers emerging as a highly effective natural remedy to address high blood pressure with clinical validation now supporting its use, these powerful heart-healthy flowers have the ability to impact many lives.

Maintaining healthy blood pressure levels is vital for our heart health. In the American Heart Association's Heart and Stroke Statistics 2019 Update, Ivor J. Benjamin, MD, president of the association, reported: "Research has shown that eliminating high blood pressure could have a larger impact on CVD deaths than the elimination of all other risk factors among women and all except smoking among men."

Research shows that approximately 80 percent of all

cardiovascular disease can be prevented by controlling high blood pressure, diabetes, and clogged arteries, along with adopting healthy lifestyle behaviors, such as not smoking and maintaining a healthy weight. I hope this book explained why and gave you a better understanding of why chronic inflammation, oxidative stress, and AGE damage, which are greatly increased in obesity, diabetes, and even in smoking, are the main contributing causes of damage to the heart and the development of most heart diseases. More importantly, I hope readers learn that these contributing causes are treatable and natural plant compounds, like those found in hibiscus flowers, can be one of the most important natural treatments.

The main goal of this book is to provide vital information to consumers so that they can learn about hibiscus flowers and how to use them effectively to positively affect their heart and their health. That a safe and natural solution exists that can not only lower blood pressure, but also address some of the most important underlying contributing causes and risk factors of most heart diseases is truly important information to share!

References

This reference list was complete the day it was compiled; however, new studies are frequently published on this important medicinal plant. The citations below are listed in chronological order with the newest research listed first. Visit www.pubmed. gov to access the latest studies cataloged at the U.S. National Library of Medicine (PubMed). *The citations appearing in bold print in this section are studies performed in humans.*

Anti-Aging and Anti-AGE Actions

Li, J., et al. "Reverse UVB-induced photoaging by *Hibiscus sabdariffa* calyx aqueous extract." *J. Sci. Food Agric.* 2019 Oct 3. (ahead of print)

Koch, K., et al. "*Hibiscus sabdariffa* L. extract prolongs lifespan and protects against amyloid-β toxicity in *Caenorhabditis elegans*: involvement of the FoxO and Nrf2 orthologues DAF-16 and SKN-1." *Eur. J. Nutr.* 2019 Feb 1. (ahead of print)

Kam, A., et al. "Plant-derived mitochondria-targeting cysteine-rich peptide modulates cellular bioenergetics." *J. Biol. Chem.* 2019 Mar; 294(11): 4000–4011.

Addor, F., et al. "Improvement of dermal parameters in aged skin after oral use of a nutrient supplement." *Clin. Cosmet. Investig. Dermatol.* 2018 Apr; 11: 195-201.

Peng, C., et al. "*Hibiscus sabdariffa* polyphenolic extract inhibits hyperglycemia, hyperlipidemia, and glycation-oxidative stress while improving insulin resistance." *J. Agric. Food Chem.* 2011 Sep 28; 59(18): 9901–9.

Brunold, C., et al. "Polysaccharides from *Hibiscus sabdariffa* flowers stimulate proliferation and differentiation of human keratinocytes." *Planta Med*. 2004 Apr; 70(4): 3703.

Anti-Atherosclerotic Actions (Prevents clogged arteries)

Yang, X., et al. "Oxidative stress-mediated atherosclerosis: mechanisms and therapies." *Front. Physiol*. 2017 Aug; 8: 600.

Goncharov, N., et al. "Reactive oxygen species in pathogenesis of atherosclerosis." *Curr. Pharm. Des*. 2015; 21(9): 1134–46.

Chen, C., et al. "Oxidized low-density lipoprotein contributes to atherogenesis via co-activation of macrophages and mast cells." *PLoS ONE*. 2015; 10: e0123088.

Wolf, D., et al. "Inflammatory mechanisms in atherosclerosis." *Hamostaseologie*. 2014; 34: 63–71.

Galkina, E., et al. "Immune and inflammatory mechanisms of atherosclerosis (*)." *Annu. Rev. Immunol*. 2009; 27: 165–97.

Kim, J., et al. "Association of age-related changes in circulating intermediary lipid metabolites, inflammatory and oxidative stress markers, and arterial stiffness in middle-aged men." *Age*. 2013; 35: 1507–19.

Chen, J. et al. "Autophagic effects of *Hibiscus sabdariffa* leaf polyphenols and epicatechin gallate (ECG) against oxidized LDL-induced injury of human endothelial cells." *Eur. J. Nutr*. 2017 Aug; 56(5): 1963–1981.

Reis, J., et al. "Action mechanism and cardiovascular effect of anthocyanins: a systematic review of animal and human studies." *J. Translational Med*. 2016 Dec; 14(35): 1–16.

Loo, S., et al. "Identification and characterization of roseltide, a knottin-type neutrophil elastase inhibitor derived from *Hibiscus sabdariffa*." *Sci Rep*. 2016 Dec; 6: 39401.

Aboonabi, A., et al. "Chemopreventive role of anthocyanins in atherosclerosis via activation of Nrf2–ARE as an indicator and modulator of redox." *Biomed. Pharma*. 2015 May; 72: 30–36.

Zhu, Y., et al. "Anti-inflammatory effect of purified dietary anthocyanin in adults with hypercholesterolemia: A randomized controlled trial." *Nutr. Metabol. Cardio. Dis*. 2013; 23(9): 843–849.

Lin, H., et al. "Chemopreventive properties and molecular mechanisms of the bioactive compounds in *Hibiscus sabdariffa* Linne." *Curr. Med. Chem*. 2011; 18(8): 1245–54.

References

Kao, E., et al. "Anthocyanin extracted from Hibiscus attenuate oxidized LDL-mediated foam cell formation involving regulation of CD36 gene." *Chem. Biol. Interact.* 2009 May; 179(2-3): 212–8.

Lo, C., et al. "Effect of Hibiscus anthocyanins-rich extract induces apoptosis of proliferating smooth muscle cell via activation of P38 MAPK and p53 pathway." *Mol. Nutr. Food Res.* 2007 Dec; 51(12): 1452–60.

Chang, Y., et al. "Hibiscus anthocyanins-rich extract inhibited LDL oxidation and oxLDL-mediated macrophages apoptosis." *Food Chem.Toxicol.* 2006 Jul; 44(7): 1015–1023.

Chen, C., et al., "Inhibitory effects of *Hibiscus sabdariffa* L extract on low-density lipoprotein oxidation and anti-hyperlipidemia in fructose-fed and cholesterol-fed rats." *J. Sci. Food Agr.* 2004. 84(15): 1989–1996.

Chen, C., et al. "*Hibiscus sabdariffa* extract inhibits the development of atherosclerosis in cholesterol-fed rabbits." *J. Agric. Food Chem.* 2003 Aug; 51(18): 5472–7.

Anti-inflammatory and Pain-Relieving Actions

Jabeur, I., et al. "Exploring the chemical and bioactive properties of *Hibiscus sabdariffa* L. calyces from Guinea-Bissau (West Africa)." *Food Funct.* 2019 Apr; 10(4): 2234–2243.

Bayani, G., et al. "Anti-inflammatory effects of *Hibiscus sabdariffa* Linn. on the IL-1β/IL-1ra ratio in plasma and hippocampus of overtrained rats and correlation with spatial memory." *Kobe J. Med. Sci.* 2018 Oct; 64(2): E73–E83.

Chou, S., et al. "Exploring the effect and mechanism of *Hibiscus sabdariffa* on urinary tract infection and experimental renal inflammation." *J. Ethnopharmacol.* 2016 Dec; 194: 617–625.

Shen, C., et al. "Anti-inflammatory activities of essential oil isolated from the calyx of *Hibiscus sabdariffa* L." *Food Funct.* 2016 Oct; 7(10): 4451–4459.

Ezzat, S., et al. "Metabolic profile and hepatoprotective activity of the anthocyanin-rich extract of *Hibiscus sabdariffa* calyces." *Pharm. Biol.* 2016 Dec; 54(12): 3172–3181.

Sogo, T., et al. "Anti-inflammatory activity and molecular mechanism of delphinidin 3-sambubioside, a Hibiscus anthocyanin." *Biofactors.* 2015 Jan-Feb; 41(1): 58–65.

Joven, J., et al. "*Hibiscus sabdariffa* extract lowers blood pressure and

improves endothelial function." *Mol. Nutr. Food Res.* 2014 Jun; 58(6): 1374–8.

Ali, M., et al. "Antinociceptive, anti-inflammatory and antidiarrheal activities of ethanolic calyx extract of *Hibiscus sabdariffa* Linn. (Malvaceae) in mice." *Zhong Xi Yi Jie He Xue Bao.* 2011 Jun; 9(6): 626–31.

Beltran-Debon, R., et al. "The aqueous extract of *Hibiscus sabdariffa* calices modulates the production of monocyte chemoattractant protein-1 in humans." *Phytomedicine.* 2010 Mar; 17(3-4): 186–91.

Kao, E., et al. "Polyphenols extracted from *Hibiscus sabdariffa* L. inhibited lipopolysaccharide-induced inflammation by improving antioxidative conditions and regulating cyclooxygenase-2 expression." *Biosci. Biotechnol. Biochem.* 2009 Feb; 73(2): 385–90.

Dafallah, A., et al. "Investigation of the anti-inflammatory activity of *Acacia nilotica* and *Hibiscus sabdariffa*." *Am. J. Chin. Med.* 1996; 24(3-4): 263–9.

Antimicrobial Actions (kills bacteria, fungi, and viruses)

Abdel-Shafi, S., et al. "Antimicrobial activity and chemical constitution of the crude, phenolic-rich extracts of *Hibiscus sabdariffa, Brassica oleracea* and *Beta vulgaris*." *Molecules.* 2019 Nov 24; 24(23).

Akarca, G., et al. "Determination of sensitivity of some food pathogens to spice extracts." *J. Food Sci. Technol.* 2019 Dec; 56(12): 5253–5261.

Takeda, Y., et al. "Antiviral activities of *Hibiscus sabdariffa* L. tea extract against human Influenza A virus rely largely on acidic pH but partially on a low-pH-independent mechanism." *Food Environ. Virol.* 2019 Oct 16. (ahead of print)

Jabeur, I., et al. "Exploring the chemical and bioactive properties of *Hibiscus sabdariffa* L. calyces from Guinea-Bissau (West Africa)." *Food Funct.* 2019 Apr; 10(4): 2234–2243.

Mohamed-Salem, R., et al. "Aqueous extract of *Hibiscus sabdariffa* inhibits pedestal induction by enteropathogenic *E. coli* and promotes bacterial filamentation *in vitro*." *PLoS One.* 2019 Mar; 14(3): e0213580.

Villasante, J., et al. "Effects of pecan nut (*Carya illinoiensis*) and roselle flower (*Hibiscus sabdariffa*) as antioxidant and antimicrobial agents for sardines (*Sardina pilchardus*)." *Molecules.* 2018 Dec; 24(1): E85.

Gonelimali, F., et al. "Antimicrobial properties and mechanism of action

References

of some plant extracts against food pathogens and spoilage microorganisms." *Front. Microbiol.* 2018 Jul; 9: 1639.

Cai, T., et al. "L-Methionine associated with *Hibiscus sabdariffa* and *Boswellia serrata* extracts are not inferior to antibiotic treatment for symptoms relief in patients affected by recurrent uncomplicated urinary tract infections: Focus on antibiotic-sparing approach." *Arch. Ital. Urol. Androl.* 2018 Jun; 90(2): 97–100.

Keramagi, A., et al. "Prediction of binding potential of natural leads against the prioritized drug targets of chikungunya and dengue viruses by computational screening." *Biotech.* 2018 Jun; 8(6): 274.

Rangel-Vargas, E., "Behavior of 11 foodborne bacteria on whole and cut mangoes var. Ataulfo and Kent and antibacterial activities of *Hibiscus sabdariffa* extracts and chemical sanitizers directly onto mangoes contaminated with foodborne bacteria." *J. Food Prot.* 2018 May; 81(5): 743–753.

Khan, Z., et al. "Green synthesis of zero-valent Fe-nanoparticles: Catalytic degradation of rhodamine B, interactions with bovine serum albumin and their enhanced antimicrobial activities." *J. Photochem. Photobiol B.* 2018 Mar; 180: 259–267.

Gomez-Aldapa, C., "Antibacterial activities of *Hibiscus sabdariffa* extracts and chemical sanitizers directly on green leaves contaminated with foodborne pathogens." *J. Food Prot.* 2018 Feb; 81(2): 209–217.

Hassan, S., et al. "Biological evaluation and molecular docking of protocatechuic acid from *Hibiscus sabdariffa* L. as a potent urease inhibitor by an ESI-MS based method." *Molecules.* 2017 Oct; 22(10): E1696.

Jabeur, I., et al. "*Hibiscus sabdariffa* L. as a source of nutrients, bioactive compounds and colouring agents." *Food Res. Int.* 2017 Oct; 100(Pt 1): 717–723.

Hassan, S., et al. "*Hibiscus sabdariffa* L. and its bioactive constituents exhibit antiviral activity against HSV-2 and anti-enzymatic properties against urease by an ESI-MS based assay." *Molecules.* 2017 Apr; 22(5): E722.

Passaro, M., et al. "Effect of a food supplement containing l-methionine on urinary tract infections in pregnancy: a prospective, multicenter observational study." *J. Altern. Complement.* Med. 2017 Jun; 23(6): 471–478.

Fauziyah, P., et al. "Combination effect of antituberculosis drugs and ethanolic extract of selected medicinal plants against multi-drug resistant *Mycobacterium tuberculosis* isolates." *Sci. Pharm.* 2017 Mar 20; 85(1): E14.

Guglietta, A. "Recurrent urinary tract infections in women: risk factors, etiology, pathogenesis and prophylaxis." *Future Microbiol.* 2017 Mar; 12: 239–246.

Chou, S., et al. "Exploring the effect and mechanism of *Hibiscus sabdariffa* on urinary tract infection and experimental renal inflammation." *J. Ethnopharmacol.* 2016 Dec; 194: 617–625.

Abdallah, E., et al. "Antibacterial efficiency of the Sudanese Roselle (*Hibiscus sabdariffa* L.), a famous beverage from Sudanese folk medicine." *J. Intercult. Ethnopharmacol.* 2016 Mar; 5(2): 186–90.

Sulistyani, H., et al. "Effect of roselle calyx extract on in vitro viability and biofilm formation ability of oral pathogenic bacteria." *Asian Pac. J. Trop. Med.* 2016 Feb; 9(2): 119–24.

D'Souza, D., et al. "Aqueous extracts of *Hibiscus sabdariffa* calyces to control Aichi virus." *Food Environ. Virol.* 2016 Jun; 8(2): 112–9.

Hassan, S., et al. "*In vitro* synergistic effect of *Hibiscus sabdariffa* aqueous extract in combination with standard antibiotics against *Helicobacter pylori* clinical isolates." *Pharm. Biol.* 2016 Sep; 54(9): 1736–40.

Gutierrez-Alcantara, E., et al. "Antibacterial effect of roselle extracts (*Hibiscus sabadariffa*), sodium hypochlorite and acetic acid against multi-drug-resistant *Salmonella* strains isolated from tomatoes." *Lett. Appl. Microbiol.* 2016 Feb; 62(2): 177–84.

Chandra Shekar, B., et al. "Herbal extracts in oral health care - A review of the current scenario and its future needs." *Pharmacogn. Rev.* 2015 Jul-Dec; 9(18): 87–92.

Joshi, S., et al. "Aqueous extracts of *Hibiscus sabdariffa* calyces decrease Hepatitis A Virus and Human Norovirus surrogate Titers." *Food Environ. Virol.* 2015 Dec; 7(4): 366–73.

Alshami, I., et al. "*Hibiscus sabdariffa* extract inhibits in vitro biofilm formation capacity of *Candida albicans* isolated from recurrent urinary tract infections." *Asian Pac. J. Trop. Biomed.* 2014 Feb; 4(2): 104–8.

Sultan, F., et al. "Chromatographic separation and identification of many fatty acids from flowers of *Hibiscus sabdariffa* L. and its inhibitory effect on some pathogenic bacteria." IJRRAS. 2014 May; 19(2): 140–149.

Higginbotham, K., et al. "Antimicrobial activity of *Hibiscus sabdariffa* aqueous extracts against *Escherichia coli* O157:H7 and *Staphylococcus aureus* in a microbiological medium and milk of various fat concentrations." *J. Food Prot.* 2014 Feb; 77(2): 262–8.

References

Builders, P., et al. "Wound healing potential of formulated extract from *Hibiscus sabdariffa* calyx." *Indian J. Pharm. Sci.* 2013 Jan; 75(1): 45–52.

Jung, E., et al. "Physicochemical properties and antimicrobial activity of Roselle (*Hibiscus sabdariffa* L.)." *J. Sci. Food Agric.* 2013 Dec; 93(15): 3769–76.

Fullerton, M., et al. "Determination of antimicrobial activity of sorrel (*Hibiscus sabdariffa*) on *Escherichia coli* O157:H7 isolated from food, veterinary, and clinical samples." *J. Med. Food.* 2011 Sep; 14(9): 950–6.

Afolabi, O., et al. "Susceptibility of cariogenic *Streptococcus mutans* to extracts of *Garcinia kola*, *Hibiscus sabdariffa*, and *Solanum americanum*." *West Afr. J. Med.* 2008 Oct; 27(4): 230–3.

Rukayadi, Y., et al. "Screening of Thai medicinal plants for anticandidal activity." *Mycoses.* 2008 Jul; 51(4): 308–12.

Anti-Obesity and Weight-Loss Actions

Diez-Echava, P., et al. "The prebiotic properties of *Hibiscus sabdariffa* extract contribute to the beneficial effects in diet-induced obesity in mice." *Food Res. Int.* 2020 Jan; 127: 108722.

Ojulari, O., et al. "Beneficial effects of natural bioactive compounds from *Hibiscus sabdariffa* L. on obesity." *Molecules.* 2019 Jan; 24(1): E210.

Morales-Luna, E., "The main beneficial effect of roselle (*Hibiscus sabdariffa*) on obesity is not only related to its anthocyanin content." *J. Sci. Food Agric.* 2019 Jan; 99(2): 596–605.

Rasheed, D., et al. "Comparative analysis of *Hibiscus sabdariffa* (roselle) hot and cold extracts in respect to their potential for α-glucosidase inhibition." *Food Chem.* 2018 Jun; 250: 236–244.

Rodriguez-Perez, C., et al. "Phenolic compounds as natural and multifunctional anti-obesity agents: A review." *Crit. Rev. Food Sci. Nutr.* 2019; 59(8): 1212–1229.

Herranz-Lopez, M., et al. "Multi-targeted molecular effects of *Hibiscus sabdariffa* polyphenols: an opportunity for a global approach to obesity." *Nutrients.* 2017 Aug; 9(8): E907.

Inrahim, K., et al. "The response of male and female rats to a high-fructose diet during adolescence following early administration of *Hibiscus sabdariffa* aqueous calyx extracts." *J. Dev. Orig. Health Dis.* 2017 Dec; 8(6): 628—637.

Gamboa-Gomez, C., "Plants with potential use on obesity and its complications." *EXCLI J.* 2015 Jul; 14: 809–31.

Buchholz, T., et al. "Medicinal plants traditionally used for treatment of obesity and diabetes mellitus - screening for pancreatic lipase and α-amylase inhibition." *Phytother. Res.* 2016 Feb; 30(2): 260–6.

Cercato, L., et al. "A systematic review of medicinal plants used for weight loss in Brazil: Is there potential for obesity treatment?" *J. Ethnopharmacol.* 2015 Dec; 176: 286–96.

Kao, E., et al. "Polyphenolic extract from *Hibiscus sabdariffa* reduces body fat by inhibiting hepatic lipogenesis and preadipocyte adipogenesis." *Food Funct.* 2016 Jan; 7(1): 171–82.

Huang, T., et al. "Effect of *Hibiscus sabdariffa* extract on high fat diet-induced obesity and liver damage in hamsters." *Food Nutr. Res.* 2015 Oct; 59: 29018.

Beltran-Debon, R., et al. "The acute impact of polyphenols from *Hibiscus sabdariffa* in metabolic homeostasis: an approach combining metabolomics and gene-expression analyses." *Food Funct.* 2015 Sep; 6(9): 2957–66.

Chang, H., et al. "*Hibiscus sabdariffa* extract inhibits obesity and fat accumulation, and improves liver steatosis in humans." *Food Funct.* 2014 Apr; 5(4): 734–9.

Villalpando-Arteaga, E., et al. "*Hibiscus sabdariffa* L. aqueous extract attenuates hepatic steatosis through down-regulation of PPAR-γ and SREBP-1c in diet-induced obese mice." *Food Funct.* 2013 Apr; 4(4): 618–26.

Ademiluyi, A., et al. "Aqueous extracts of Roselle (*Hibiscus sabdariffa* Linn.) varieties inhibit α-amylase and α-glucosidase activities *in vitro*." *J. Med. Food.* 2013 Jan; 16(1): 88–93.

Adisakwattana, S., et al. "*In vitro* inhibitory effects of plant-based foods and their combinations on intestinal α-glucosidase and pancreatic α-amylase." *BMC Complement. Altern Med.* 2012 Jul; 12: 110.

Herranz-Lopez, M., et al. "Synergism of plant-derived polyphenols in adipogenesis: perspectives and implications." *Phytomedicine.* 2012 Feb; 19(3-4): 253–61.

Carvajal-Zarrabal, O., "Effect of *Hibiscus sabdariffa* L. dried calyx ethanol extract on fat absorption-excretion, and body weight implication in rats." *J. Biomed. Biotechnol.* 2009; 2009: 394592.

Kim, J., et al. "*Hibiscus sabdariffa* L. water extract inhibits the adipocyte differentiation through the PI3-K and MAPK pathway." *J. Ethnopharmacol.* 2007 Nov; 114(2): 260–7.

Alarcon-Aguilar, F., et al. "Effect of *Hibiscus sabdariffa* on obesity in MSG mice." *J. Ethnopharmacol.* 2007 Oct; 114(1): 66–71.

Kim, M., et al. "Hibiscus extract inhibits the lipid droplet accumulation and adipogenic transcription factors expression of 3T3-L1 preadipocytes." *J. Altern. Complement. Med.* 2003 Aug; 9(4): 499–504.

Hansawasdi, C., et al. "Alpha-amylase inhibitors from roselle (*Hibiscus sabdariffa* Linn.) tea." *Biosci. Biotechnol. Biochem.* 2000 May; 64(5): 1041-3.

Anti-Osteoporotic Actions

Fernandez-Arroyo, S., et al. "The impact of polyphenols on chondrocyte growth and survival: a preliminary report." *Food Nutr. Res.* 2015 Oct; 59: 29311.

Antioxidant Actions

Das, A., et al. "Synergistic effect of herbal plant extract (*Hibiscus sabdariffa*) in maintain the antioxidant activity of decaffeinated green tea from various parts of Assam." *J. Food Sci. Technol.* 2019 Nov; 56(11): 5009–5016.

Zihad, S., et al. "Nutritional value, micronutrient and antioxidant capacity of some green leafy vegetables commonly used by southern coastal people of Bangladesh." *Heliyon.* 2019 Nov; 5(11): e02768.

Si, L., et al. "Roselle attenuates cardiac hypertrophy after myocardial infarction *in vivo* and *in vitro*." *EXCLI J.* 2019 Sep; 18: 876–892.

Thien, V., et al. "A new lignan from the flowers of *Hibiscus sabdariffa* L. (Malvaceae)." *Nat. Prod. Res.* 2019 Sep; 23: 1–6.

Gerald, C., et al. "Sorrel extract reduces oxidant production in airway epithelial cells exposed to swine barn dust extract *in vitro*." *Mediators Inflamm.* 2019 Aug; 2019: 7420468.

Perez-Torres, I., et al. "Myocardial protection from ischemia-reperfusion damage by the antioxidant effect of *Hibiscus sabdariffa* Linnaeus on metabolic syndrome rats." *Oxid. Med. Cell. Longev.* 2019 Mar; 2019: 1724194.

Adeyemi, D., et al. "*Hibiscus sabdariffa* renews pancreatic β-cells in experimental type 1 diabetic model rats." *Morphologie.* 2019 Jun; 103(341 Pt 2): 80–93.

Pengkumsri, N., et al. "Influence of extraction methods on total phenolic content and antioxidant properties of some of the commonly used plants in Thailand." *Pak. J. Biol. Sci.* 2019 Jan; 22(3): 117–126.

Jabeur, I., et al. "Exploring the chemical and bioactive properties of *Hibiscus sabdariffa* L. calyces from Guinea-Bissau (West Africa)." *Food Funct.* 2019 Apr; 10(4): 2234–2243.

Ochoa-Velasco, C., et al. "Mass transfer modeling of the antioxidant extraction of roselle flower (*Hibiscus sabdariffa*)." *J. Food Sci. Technol.* 2019 Feb; 56(2): 1008–1015.

Piovensana, A., et al. "Composition analysis of carotenoids and phenolic compounds and antioxidant activity from hibiscus calyces (*Hibiscus sabdariffa* L.) by HPLC-DAD-MS/MS." *Phytochem. Anal.* 2019 Mar; 30(2): 208–217.

Nurkhasanah, N., et al. "The increasing of catalase activity in dimethyl-benz-α-anthracene (DMBA) induced rat treated by *Hibiscus sabdariffa* L extract." *Pak. J. Pharm. Sci.* 2018 May; 31(3): 849–856.

Pimentel-Moral, S., et al. "Development and stability evaluation of water-in-edible oils emulsions formulated with the incorporation of hydrophilic *Hibiscus sabdariffa* extract." *Food Chem.* 2018 Sep; 260: 200–207.

Famurewa, A., et al. "Abrogation of hepatic damage induced by anticancer drug methotrexate by zobo (*Hibiscus sabdariffa* extract) supplementation via targeting oxidative hepatotoxicity in rats." *J. Diet. Suppl.* 2019; 16(3): 318–330.

Maciel, L., et al. "*Hibiscus sabdariffa* anthocyanins-rich extract: Chemical stability, *in vitro* antioxidant and antiproliferative activities." *Food Chem. Toxicol.* 2018 Mar; 113: 187–197.

Hosseini, A., et al. "Protective effect of *Hibiscus sabdariffa* on doxorubicin-induced cytotoxicity in H9c2 cardiomyoblast cells." *Iran J. Pharm. Res.* 2017 Spring; 16(2): 708–713.

Subhaswaraj, P., et al. "Determination of antioxidant activity of *Hibiscus sabdariffa* and *Croton caudatus* in *Saccharomyces cerevisiae* model system." *J. Food Sci. Technol.* 2017 Aug; 54(9): 2728–2736.

Nguyen, N., et al. "Polyphenols reported to shift APAP-induced changes in MAPK signaling and toxicity outcomes." *Chem. Biol. Interact.* 2017 Nov; 277: 129–136.

Hadi, A., et al. "The effect of green tea and sour tea (*Hibiscus sabdariffa* L.) supplementation on oxidative stress and muscle damage in athletes." *J. Diet. Suppl.* 2017 May; 14(3): 346–357.

References

Jabeur, I., et al. "*Hibiscus sabdariffa* L. as a source of nutrients, bioactive compounds and colouring agents." *Food Res. Int.* 2017 Oct; 100(Pt 1): 717–723.

Nazratun Nafizah, A., et al. "Aqueous calyxes extract of Roselle or *Hibiscus sabdariffa* Linn supplementation improves liver morphology in streptozotocin induced diabetic rats." *Arab. J. Gastroenterol.* 2017 Mar; 18(1): 13–20.

Kapepula, P., et al. "Comparison of metabolic profiles and bioactivities of the leaves of three edible Congolese *Hibiscus* species." *Nat. Prod. Res.* 2017 Dec; 31(24): 2885–2892.

Ogundele, O., et al. "Development of functional beverages from blends of *Hibiscus sabdariffa* extract and selected fruit juices for optimal antioxidant properties." *Food Sci. Nutr.* 2016 Jan; 4(5): 679–85.

Ezzat, S., et al. "Metabolic profile and hepatoprotective activity of the anthocyanin-rich extract of *Hibiscus sabdariffa* calyces." *Pharm. Biol.* 2016 Dec; 54(12): 3172–3181.

Soto, M., et al. "Infusion of *Hibiscus sabdariffa* L. modulates oxidative stress in patients with Marfan Syndrome." *Mediators Inflamm.* 2016; 2016: 8625203.

Bi, W., et al. "Investigation of free amino acid, total phenolics, antioxidant activity and purine alkaloids to assess the health properties of non-Camellia tea." *Acta Pharm. Sin. B.* 2016 Mar; 6(2): 170–81.

Rodriguez-Ramiro, I., "Polyphenols and non-alcoholic fatty liver disease: impact and mechanisms." *Proc. Nutr. Soc.* 2016 Feb; 75(1): 47–60.

Grajeda-Iglesias, C., et al. "Antioxidant activity of protocatechuates evaluated by DPPH, ORAC, and CAT methods." *Food Chem.* 2016 Mar; 194: 749–57.

Formagio, A., et al. "Phenolic compounds of *Hibiscus sabdariffa* and influence of organic residues on its antioxidant and antitumoral properties." *Braz. J. Biol.* 2015 Jan–Mar; 75(1): 69–76.

Joven, J., et al. "*Hibiscus sabdariffa* extract lowers blood pressure and improves endothelial function." *Mol. Nutr. Food Res.* 2014 Jun; 58(6): 1374–8.

Lin, H., et al. "Antioxidant effects of 14 Chinese traditional medicinal herbs against human low-density lipoprotein oxidation." *J. Tradit. Complement. Med.* 2014 Nov; 5(1): 51–5.

Abdul Hamid, Z., et al. "The role of *Hibiscus sabdariffa* L. (Roselle) in maintenance of *ex vivo* murine bone marrow-derived hematopoietic stem cells." *Sci. World J.* 2014; 2014: 258192.

Victor, E., et al. "Efficacy of *Hibiscus sabdariffa* and *Telfairia occidentalis* in the attenuation of CCl4-mediated oxidative stress." *Asian Pac. J. Trop. Med.* 2014 Sep; 7S1: S321–6.

Adeyemi, D., et al. "Anti-hepatotoxic activities of *Hibiscus sabdariffa* L. in animal model of streptozotocin diabetes-induced liver damage." *BMC Complement. Altern. Med.* 2014 Jul 30; 14: 277.

Sarkar, B., et al. "Antioxidant and DNA damage protective properties of anthocyanin-rich extracts from *Hibiscus* and *Ocimum*: a comparative study." *Nat. Prod. Res.* 2014; 28(17): 1393–8.

Ademiluyi, A., et al. "Anthocyanin - rich red dye of *Hibiscus sabdariffa* calyx modulates cisplatin-induced nephrotoxicity and oxidative stress in rats." *Int. J. Biomed. Sci.* 2013 Dec; 9(4): 243–8.

Mohamed, J., et al. "The protective effect of aqueous extracts of roselle (*Hibiscus sabdariffa* L. UKMR-2) against red blood cell membrane oxidative stress in rats with streptozotocin-induced diabetes." *Clinics* (Sao Paulo). 2013 Oct; 68(10): 1358–63.

Fernandez-Arroyo, S., et al. "Bioavailability study of a polyphenol-enriched extract from *Hibiscus sabdariffa* in rats and associated antioxidant status." *Mol. Nutr. Food Res.* 2012 Oct; 56(10): 1590–5.

Frank, T., et al. "Consumption of *Hibiscus sabdariffa* L. aqueous extract and its impact on systemic antioxidant potential in healthy subjects." *J. Sci. Food Agric.* 2012 Aug 15; 92(10): 2207–18.

Okoko, T., et al. "*Hibiscus sabdariffa* extractivities on cadmium-mediated alterations of human U937 cell viability and activation." *Asian Pac. J. Trop. Med.* 2012 Jan; 5(1): 33–6.

Ajiboye, T., et al. "Antioxidant and drug detoxification potentials of *Hibiscus sabdariffa* anthocyanin extract." *Drug Chem. Toxicol.* 2011 Apr; 34(2):109–15.

Ochani, P., et al. "Antioxidant and antihyperlipidemic activity of *Hibiscus sabdariffa* Linn. leaves and calyces extracts in rats." *Indian J. Exp. Biol.* 2009 Apr; 47(4): 276–82.

Umar, I., et al. "The effect of aqueous extracts of *Hibiscus sabdariffa* (Sorrel) calyces on heamatological profile and organ pathological changes in

References

Trypanasoma congolense - infected rats." *Afr. J. Tradit. Complement. Altern Med.* 2009 Jul; 6(4): 585–91.

Sayago-Ayerdi, S., et al. "Dietary fiber content and associated antioxidant compounds in Roselle flower (*Hibiscus sabdariffa* L.) beverage." *J. Agric. Food Chem.* 2007 Sep; 55(19): 7886-90.

Hirunpanich, V., et al. "Hypocholesterolemic and antioxidant effects of aqueous extracts from the dried calyx of *Hibiscus sabdariffa* L. in hypercholesterolemic rats." *J. Ethnopharmacol.* 2006 Jan; 103(2): 252–60.

Amin, A, et al. "Effects of Roselle and Ginger on cisplatin-induced reproductive toxicity in rats." *Asian J. Androl.* 2006 Sep; 8(5): 607–12.

Farombi, E., et al. "Free radical scavenging and antigenotoxic activities of natural phenolic compounds in dried flowers of *Hibiscus sabdariffa* L." *Mol. Nutr. Food Res.* 2005 Dec; 49(12): 1120—8.

Hirunpanich, V., et. al. "Antioxidant effects of aqueous extracts from dried calyx of *Hibiscus sabdariffa* Linn. (Roselle) *in vitro* using rat low-density lipoprotein (LDL)." *Biol. Pharm. Bull.* 2005 Mar; 28(3): 481–4.

Adetutu, A., et al. "Anticlastogenic effects of *Hibiscus sabdariffa* fruits against sodium arsenite-induced micronuclei formation in erythrocytes in mouse bone marrow." *Phytother. Res.* 2004 Oct;18(10): 862–4.

Suboh, S., et al. "Protective effects of selected medicinal plants against protein degradation, lipid peroxidation and deformability loss of oxidatively stressed human erythrocytes." *Phytother. Res.* 2004 Apr; 18(4): 280–4.

Anti-spasmodic Actions

Fouda, A., et al. "Inhibitory effects of aqueous extract of *Hibiscus sabdariffa* on contractility of the rat bladder and uterus." *Can. J. Physiol. Pharmacol.* 2007 Oct; 85(10): 1020–31.

Ali, M., et al. "Investigation of the antispasmodic potential of *Hibiscus sabdariffa* calyces." *J. Ethnopharmacol.* 1991 Feb; 31(2): 249—57.

Blood Pressure–Lowering Actions

Najafpour Noushehri, S., et al. "The efficacy of sour tea (*Hibiscus sabdariffa* L.) on selected cardiovascular disease risk factors: A systematic review and meta-analysis of randomized clinical trials." *Phytother. Res.* 2020 Jan 14. (ahead of print)

Al-Anbaki, M., et al. "Treating uncontrolled hypertension with *Hibiscus sabdariffa* when standard treatment is insufficient: pilot intervention." *J. Altern. Complement. Med.* 2019 Oct 10. (ahead of print)

Nurfaradilla S., et al. "Effects of *Hibiscus sabdariffa* calyces aqueous extract on the antihypertensive potency of captopril in the two-kidney-one-clip rat hypertension model." *Evid. Based Complement. Alternat. Med.* 2019 Jul; 2019: 9694212.

Jalalyazdi, M., et al. "Effect of *Hibiscus sabdariffa* on blood pressure in patients with stage 1 hypertension." *J. Adv. Pharm. Technol. Res.* 2019 Jul-Sep; 10(3): 107–111.

Zheoat, A., et al. "Hibiscus acid from *Hibiscus sabdariffa* (Malvaceae) has a vasorelaxant effect on the rat aorta. *Fitoterapia*. 2019 Apr; 134: 5–13.

Seck, S., et al. "Clinical efficacy of African traditional medicines in hypertension: A randomized controlled trial with *Combretum micranthum* and *Hibiscus sabdariffa*." *J. Hum. Hypertens.* 2017 Dec; 32(1): 75–81.

Abdel-Rahman, R., et al. "Antihypertensive effects of roselle-olive combination in L-NAME-induced hypertensive rats." *Oxid. Med. Cell. Longev.* 2017; 2017: 9460653.

Kafeshani, M., et al. "A comparative study of the effect of green tea and sour tea on blood pressure and lipid profile in healthy adult men." *ARYA Atheroscler.* 2017 May; 13(3): 109–116.

Nwachukwu, D., et al. "Does consumption of an aqueous extract of *Hibiscus sabdariffa* affect renal function in subjects with mild to moderate hypertension?" *J. Physiol. Sci.* 2017 Jan; 67(1): 227–234.

Micucci, M., "*Hibiscus sabdariffa* L. flowers and *Olea europea* L. leaves extract-based formulation for hypertension care: *in vitro* efficacy and toxicological profile." *J. Med. Food.* 2016 May; 19(5): 504–12.

Shayoub, M. "Hibiscus miracle in treatment of hypertension." *Am. J. Pharm. Tech Res.* 2016 Feb; 6(2): 293-310.

Asgary, S., et al. "Evaluation of the effects of roselle (*Hibiscus sabdariffa* L.) on oxidative stress and serum levels of lipids, insulin and hs-CRP in adult patients with metabolic syndrome: a double-blind placebo-controlled clinical trial." *J. Complement. Integr. Med.* 2016 Jun; 13(2): 175–80.

Nwachukwu, D., et al. "Effects of aqueous extract of *Hibiscus sabdariffa* on the renin-angiotensin-aldosterone system of Nigerians with mild to moderate essential hypertension: A comparative study with lisinopril." *Indian J. Pharmacol.* 2015 Sep–Oct; 47(5): 540-5.

References

Nwachukwu, D., "Effect of *Hibiscus sabdariffa* on blood pressure and electrolyte profile of mild to moderate hypertensive Nigerians: A comparative study with hydrochlorothiazide." *Niger. J. Clin. Pract.* 2015 Nov-Dec; 18(6): 762–70.

Beltran-Debon, R., et al. "The acute impact of polyphenols from *Hibiscus sabdariffa* in metabolic homeostasis: an approach combining metabolomics and gene-expression analyses." *Food Funct.* 2015 Sep; 6(9): 2957–66.

Serban, C., et al. "Effect of sour tea (*Hibiscus sabdariffa* L.) on arterial hypertension: a systematic review and meta-analysis of randomized controlled trials." *J. Hypertens.* 2015 Jun; 33(6): 1119–27.

Fernandez-Arroyo, S., et al. "Managing hypertension by polyphenols." *Planta Med.* 2015 Jun; 81(8): 624–9.

Joven, J., et al. "*Hibiscus sabdariffa* extract lowers blood pressure and improves endothelial function." *Mol. Nutr. Food Res.* 2014 Jun; 58(6): 1374–8.

Aliyu, B., et al. "The aqueous calyx extract of *Hibiscus sabdariffa* lowers blood pressure and heart rate via sympathetic nervous system dependent mechanisms." *Niger. J. Physiol. Sci.* 2014 Dec; 29(2): 131–6.

Hopkins, A., et al. "*Hibiscus sabdariffa* L. in the treatment of hypertension and hyperlipidemia: a comprehensive review of animal and human studies." *Fitoterapia.* 2013 Mar; 85: 84–94.

Mojiminiyi, F., et al. "Attenuation of salt-induced hypertension by aqueous calyx extract of *Hibiscus sabdariffa*." *Niger. J. Physiol. Sci.* 2012 Dec; 27(2): 195–200.

Mohagheghi, A., et al. "The effect of *Hibiscus sabdariffa* on lipid profile, creatinine, and serum electrolytes: a randomized clinical trial." *ISRN Gastroenterol.* 2011; 2011: 976019.

McKay, D., et al. "*Hibiscus sabdariffa* L. tea (tisane) lowers blood pressure in prehypertensive and mildly hypertensive adults." *J. Nutr.* 2010 Feb; 140(2): 298–303.

Wahabi, H., et al. "The effectiveness of *Hibiscus sabdariffa* in the treatment of hypertension: A systematic review." *Phytomedicine.* 2010; 17: 83–86.

Sarr, M., et al. "*In vitro* vasorelaxation mechanisms of bioactive compounds extracted from *Hibiscus sabdariffa* on rat thoracic aorta." *Nutr. Metab.* (Lond). 2009 Nov 2; 6: 45.

Ojeda, D., et al. "Inhibition of angiotensin convertin enzyme (ACE) activity by the anthocyanins delphinidin- and cyanidin-3-O-sambubiosides from *Hibiscus sabdariffa.*" *J. Ethnopharmacol.* 2010 Jan; 127(1): 7—10.

Mozaffari-Khosravi, H., et al. "The effects of sour tea (*Hibiscus sabdariffa*) on hypertension in patients with type II diabetes." *J. Hum. Hypertens.* 2009 Jan; 23(1): 48–54.

Mojiminiyi, F., "Antihypertensive effect of an aqueous extract of the calyx of *Hibiscus sabdariffa.*" *Fitoterapia.* 2007 Jun; 78(4): 292–7.

Herrera-Arellano, A., et al. "Clinical effects produced by a standardized herbal medicinal product of *Hibiscus sabdariffa* on patients with hypertension. A randomized, double-blind, lisinopril-controlled clinical trial." *Planta Med.* 2007 Jan; 73(1): 6–12.

Ajay, M., et al. "Mechanisms of the anti-hypertensive effect of *Hibiscus sabdariffa* L. calyces." *J. Ethnopharmacol.* 2007 Feb; 109(3): 388–93.

Mojiminiyi, F., et al. "Antihypertensive effect of an aqueous extract of the calyx of *Hibiscus sabdariffa.*" *Fitoterapia.* 2007; 78: 292–297.

Herrera-Arellano, A., "Effectiveness and tolerability of a standardized extract from *Hibiscus sabdariffa* in patients with mild to moderate hypertension: a controlled and randomized clinical trial." *Phytomedicine.* 2004 Jul; 11(5): 375–82.

Odigie, I., et al. "Chronic administration of aqueous extract of *Hibiscus sabdariffa* attenuates hypertension and reverses cardiac hypertrophy in 2K-1C hypertensive rats." *J. Ethnopharmacol.* 2003 Jun; 86(2-3): 181–5.

Onyenekwe, P., et al. "Antihypertensive effect of roselle (*Hibiscus sabdariffa*) calyx infusion in spontaneously hypertensive rats and a comparison of its toxicity with that in Wistar rats." *Cell. Biochem. Funct.* 1999 Sep; 17(3): 199–206.

Haji, R., et al. "The effect of sour tea (*Hibiscus sabdariffa*) on essential hypertension." *J. Ethnopharmacol.* 1999 Jun; 65(3): 231–6.

Adegunloye, B., "Mechanisms of the blood pressure lowering effect of the calyx extract of *Hibiscus sabdariffa* in rats." *Afr. J. Med. Med Sci.* 1996 Sep; 25(3): 235–8.

el-Saadany, S., et al. "Biochemical dynamics and hypocholesterolemic action of *Hibiscus sabdariffa* (Karkade)." *Nahrung.* 1991; 35(6): 567–76.

References

Brain Protective & Anti-Alzheimer's Actions

Koch, K., et al. *"Hibiscus sabdariffa* L. extract prolongs lifespan and protects against amyloid-β toxicity in *Caenorhabditis elegans*: involvement of the FoxO and Nrf2 orthologues DAF-16 and SKN-1." *Eur. J. Nutr.* 2019 Feb 1. (ahead of print)

Oboh, G., et al. "Phenolic constituents and inhibitory effects of *Hibiscus sabdariffa* L. (Sorrel) calyx on cholinergic, monoaminergic, and purinergic enzyme activities." *J. Diet Suppl.* 2018 Nov; 15(6): 910–922.

Owoeye, O., et al. "Evaluation of neuroprotective effect of *Hibiscus sabdariffa* Linn. aqueous extract against ischaemic-reperfusion insult by bilateral common carotid artery occlusion in adult male rats." *Niger. J. Physiol. Sci.* 2017 Jun 30; 32(1): 97–104.

Bakhtiari, E., et al. "Protective effect of *Hibiscus sabdariffa* against serum/glucose deprivation-induced PC12 cells injury." *Avicenna J. Phytomed.* 2015 May-Jun; 5(3): 231–7.

Suryanti, S., et al. "Red sorrel (*Hibiscus sabdariffa*) prevents the ethanol-induced deficits of Purkinje cells in the cerebellum." *Bratisl. Lek. Listy.* 2015; 116(2): 109–14.

Essa, M., et al. "*Hibiscus sabdariffa* affects ammonium chloride-induced hyperammonemic rats." *Evid. Based Complement. Alternat. Med.* 2007 Sep; 4(3): 321–5.

Cancer Preventative & Anti-cancer Actions

Malacrida, A., et al. "Anti-multiple myeloma potential of secondary Metabolites from *Hibiscus sabdariffa*." *Molecules*. 2019 Jul; 24(13): E2500.

Gheller, A., et al. "Antimutagenic effect of *Hibiscus sabdariffa* L. aqueous extract on rats treated with monosodium glutamate." *Scientific World Journal*. 2017; 2017: 9392532.

Tsai, T., et al. "Anthocyanins from roselle extract arrest cell cycle G2/M phase transition via ATM/Chk pathway in p53-deficient leukemia HL-60 cells." *Environ. Toxicol.* 2017 Apr; 32(4): 1290–1304.

Goldberg, K., et al. "Components in aqueous *Hibiscus rosa-sinensis* flower extract inhibit *in vitro* melanoma cell growth." *J. Tradit. Complement. Med.* 2016 Feb 23; 7(1): 45–49.

Malacrida, A., et al. "Antitumoral effect of *Hibiscus sabdariffa* on human squamous cell carcinoma and multiple myeloma cells." *Nutr. Cancer.* 2016 Oct; 68(7): 1161–70.

Amran, N., et al. "Antioxidant and cytotoxic effect of *Barringtonia racemosa* and *Hibiscus sabdariffa* fruit extracts in MCF-7 human breast cancer cell line." *Pharmacognosy Res.* 2016 Jan–Mar; 8(1): 66–70.

Formagio, A., et al. "Phenolic compounds of *Hibiscus sabdariffa* and influence of organic residues on its antioxidant and antitumoral properties." *Braz. J. Biol.* 2015 Jan–Mar; 75(1): 69–76.

Chiu, C., et al. "*Hibiscus sabdariffa* leaf polyphenolic extract induces human melanoma cell death, apoptosis, and autophagy." *J. Food Sci.* 2015 Mar; 80(3): H649–58.

Sarkar, B., et al. "Antioxidant and DNA damage protective properties of anthocyanin-rich extracts from *Hibiscus* and *Ocimum*: a comparative study." *Nat. Prod. Res.* 2014; 28(17): 1393–8.

Tsai, T., et al. "An anthocyanin-rich extract from *Hibiscus sabdariffa* Linnaeus inhibits N-nitrosomethylurea-induced leukemia in rats." *J. Agric. Food Chem.* 2014 Feb; 62(7): 1572–80.

Olvera-Garcia, V., et al. "*Hibiscus sabdariffa* L. extracts inhibit the mutagenicity in microsuspension assay and the proliferation of HeLa cells." *J. Food Sci.* 2008 Jun; 73(5): T75–81.

Lin, H., et al. "Chemopreventive properties of *Hibiscus sabdariffa* L. on human gastric carcinoma cells through apoptosis induction and JNK/p38 MAPK signaling activation." *Chem. Biol. Interact.* 2007 Jan; 165(1): 59–75.

Hou, D., et al. "Delphinidin 3-sambubioside, a *Hibiscus* anthocyanin, induces apoptosis in human leukemia cells through reactive oxygen species-mediated mitochondrial pathway." *Arch. Biochem. Biophys.* 2005 Aug; 440(1): 101–9.

Chang, Y., et al. "Hibiscus anthocyanins rich extract-induced apoptotic cell death in human promyelocytic leukemia cells." *Toxicol. Appl. Pharmacol.* 2005 Jun; 205(3): 201–12.

Lin, H., et al. "Hibiscus polyphenol-rich extract induces apoptosis in human gastric carcinoma cells via p53 phosphorylation and p38 MAPK/FasL cascade pathway." *Mol. Carcinog.* 2005 Jun; 43(2): 86–99.

Tseng, T., et al. "Induction of apoptosis by hibiscus protocatechuic acid in human leukemia cells via reduction of retinoblastoma (RB) phosphorylation and Bcl-2 expression." *Biochem. Pharmacol.* 2000 Aug; 60(3): 307–15.

References

Chewonarin, T., et al. "Effects of roselle (*Hibiscus sabdariffa* Linn.), a Thai medicinal plant, on the mutagenicity of various known mutagens in *Salmonella typhimurium* and on formation of aberrant crypt foci induced by the colon carcinogens azoxymethane and 2-amino-1-methyl-6-phenylimidazo[4,5-b]pyridine in F344 rats." *Food Chem. Toxicol.* 1999 Jun; 37(6): 591–601.

Tseng, T., et al. "Inhibitory effect of Hibiscus protocatechuic acid on tumor promotion in mouse skin." *Cancer Lett.* 1998 Apr; 126(2): 199–207.

Cholesterol-Lowering Actions

Diamond, D., and Ravnskov. U. "How statistical deception created the appearance that statins are safe and effective in primary and secondary prevention of cardiovascular disease." *Expert Review of Clinical Pharmacology.* 2015; 8 (2): 201.

Hamazaki, T., et al. "Towards a paradigm shift in cholesterol treatment. a re-examination of the cholesterol issue in Japan: Abstracts." *Ann. Nutr. Metab.* 2015; 66(suppl 4): 1–116.

Schupt, N., et al. "Relationship between plasma lipids and all-cause mortality in nondemented elderly." *J. Am. Geriatr. Soc.* 2005 Feb; 53(2): 219–26.

Linna, M., et al. "Circulating oxidised LDL lipids, when proportioned to HDL-c, emerged as a risk factor of all-cause mortality in a population-based survival study." *Age and Ageing,* 2019 Jan; 42(1): 110–113.

Hajifaraji, M., et al. "Effects of aqueous extracts of dried calyx of sour tea (*Hibiscus sabdariffa* L.) on polygenic dyslipidemia: A randomized clinical trial." *Avicenna J. Phytomed.* 2018 Jan–Feb; 8(1): 24–32.

Kafeshani, M., et al. "A comparative study of the effect of green tea and sour tea on blood pressure and lipid profile in healthy adult men." *ARYA Atheroscler.* 2017 May; 13(3): 109–116.

Showande, S., et al. "*In vivo* pharmacodynamic and pharmacokinetic interactions of *Hibiscus sabdariffa* calyces extracts with simvastatin." *J. Clin. Pharm. Ther.* 2017 Dec; 42(6): 695–703.

Jeenduang, N., et al. "APOE and CETP TaqIB polymorphisms influence metabolic responses to *Hibiscus sabdariffa* L. and *Gynostemma pentaphyllum* Makino tea consumption in hypercholesterolemic subjects. *Asia Pac. J. Clin. Nutr.* 2017 Mar; 26(2): 368–378.

Asgary, S., et al. "Evaluation of the effects of roselle (*Hibiscus sabdariffa* L.) on oxidative stress and serum levels of lipids, insulin and hs-CRP in

103

adult patients with metabolic syndrome: a double-blind placebo-controlled clinical trial." *J. Complement. Integr. Med.* 2016 Jun; 13(2): 175–80.

Ajoboye, T., et al. *"Hibiscus sabdariffa* calyx palliates insulin resistance, hyperglycemia, dyslipidemia and oxidative rout in fructose-induced metabolic syndrome rats." *J. Sci. Food Agric.* 2016 Mar; 96(5): 1522–31.

Sabzghabaee, A., "Effect of *Hibiscus sabdariffa* calices on dyslipidemia in obese adolescents: a triple-masked randomized controlled trial." *Mater. Sociomed.* 2013; 25(2): 76–9.

Chen, J., et al. *"Hibiscus sabdariffa* leaf polyphenolic extract inhibits LDL oxidation and foam cell formation involving up-regulation of LXRα/ ABCA1 pathway." *Food Chem.* 2013 Nov; 141(1): 397–406.

Hopkins, A., et al. *"Hibiscus sabdariffa* L. in the treatment of hypertension and hyperlipidemia: a comprehensive review of animal and human studies." *Fitoterapia.* 2013 Mar; 85: 84–94.

Hernandez-Perez, F., et al. "[Therapeutic use *Hibiscus sabadariffa* extract in the treatment of hypercholesterolemia. A randomized clinical trial]." *Rev. Med. Inst. Mex. Seguro. Soc.* 2011 Sep-Oct; 49(5): 469–80.

Ekor, M., et al. *"Hibiscus sabdariffa* ethanolic extract protects against dyslipidemia and oxidative stress induced by chronic cholesterol administration in rabbits." *Afr. J. Med. Med. Sci.* 2010 Dec; 39 Suppl: 161–70.

Duangjai, A., et al. "Potential mechanisms of hypocholesterolaemic effect of Thai spices/dietary extracts." *Nat. Prod. Res.* 2011 Feb; 25(4): 341–52.

Yang, M., et al. "The hypolipidemic effect of *Hibiscus sabdariffa* polyphenols via inhibiting lipogenesis and promoting hepatic lipid clearance." *J. Agric. Food Chem.* 2010 Jan; 58(2): 850–9.

Kuriyan, R., et al. "An evaluation of the hypolipidemic effect of an extract of *Hibiscus sabdariffa* leaves in hyperlipidemic Indians: a double blind, placebo controlled trial." *BMC Complement. Altern. Med.* 2010; 10: 27.

Gosain, S., et al. "Hypolipidemic effect of ethanolic extract from the leaves of *Hibiscus sabdariffa* L. in hyperlipidemic rats." *Acta Pol. Pharm.* 2010; 67: 179–184.

Ochani, P., et al. "Antioxidant and antihyperlipidemic activity of *Hibiscus sabdariffa* Linn. leaves and calyces extracts in rats." *Indian J. Exp Biol.* 2009 Apr; 47(4): 276–82.

Mozaffari-Khosravi, H., et al. "Effects of sour tea (*Hibiscus sabdariffa*) on lipid profile and lipoproteins in patients with type II diabetes." *J. Altern. Complement. Med.* 2009 Aug; 15(8): 899–903.

Farombi, E., "Hypolipidemic and antioxidant effects of ethanolic extract from dried calyx of *Hibiscus sabdariffa* in alloxan-induced diabetic rats." *Fundam. Clin. Pharmacol.* 2007 Dec; 21(6): 601–9.

Lin, T., et al. "*Hibiscus sabdariffa* extract reduces serum cholesterol in men and women." *Nutr. Res.* 2007; 27: 140–145.

Hirunpanich, V., et al. "Hypocholesterolemic and antioxidant effects of aqueous extracts from the dried calyx of *Hibiscus sabdariffa* L. in hypercholesterolemic rats." *J. Ethnopharmacol.* 2006 Jan; 103(2): 252–60.

Carvajal-Zarrabal, O., "The consumption of *Hibiscus sabdariffa* dried calyx ethanolic extract reduced lipid profile in rats." *Plant Foods Hum. Nutr.* 2005 Dec; 60(4): 153–9.

Olatunji, L., "Effects of aqueous extracts of petals of red and green *Hibiscus sabdariffa* on plasma lipid and hematological variables in rats." *Pharm. Biol.* 2005; 43: 471–474.

El-Saadany, S., et al. "Biochemical dynamics and hypocholesterolemic action of *Hibiscus sabdariffa* (Karkade)." *Nahrung.* 1991; 35: 567–576.

Detoxifying Actions

Okoko, T., et al. "*Hibiscus sabdariffa* extractivities on cadmium-mediated alterations of human U937 cell viability and activation." *Asian Pac. J. Trop. Med.* 2012 Jan; 5(1): 33–6.

Ajiboye, T., et al. "Antioxidant and drug detoxification potentials of *Hibiscus sabdariffa* anthocyanin extract." *Drug Chem. Toxicol.* 2011 Apr; 34(2):109–15.

Asagba, S., et al. "Influence of aqueous extract of *Hibiscus sabdariffa* L. petal on cadmium toxicity in rats." *Biol. Trace Elem. Res.* 2007 Jan; 115(1): 47–57.

Diabetes

Kartinah, N., et al. "The potential of *Hibiscus sabdariffa* Linn in inducing glucagon-like peptide-1 via SGLT-1 and GLPR in DM rats." *Biomed. Res. Int.* 2019 Nov; 2019: 8724824.

Alegbe, E., et al. "Antidiabetic activity-guided isolation of gallic and protocatechuic acids from *Hibiscus sabdariffa* calyxes." *J. Food Biochem.* 2019 Jul; 43(7): e12927.

Adeyemi, D., et al. "*Hibiscus sabdariffa* renews pancreatic β-cells in experimental type 1 diabetic model rats." *Morphologie*. 2019 Jun; 103(341 Pt 2): 80–93.

Giacoman-Martinez, A., et al. "Triterpenoids from *Hibiscus sabdariffa* L. with PPARδ/γ dual agonist action: *in vivo, in vitro* and in silico studies." *Planta Med*. 2019 Mar; 85(5): 412–423.

Seung, T., et al. "Ethyl acetate fraction from *Hibiscus sabdariffa* L. attenuates diabetes-associated cognitive impairment in mice." *Food Res. Int*. 2018 Mar; 105: 589–598.

Inrahim, K., et al. "The response of male and female rats to a high-fructose diet during adolescence following early administration of *Hibiscus sabdariffa* aqueous calyx extracts." *J. Dev. Orig. Health Dis*. 2017 Dec; 8(6): 628–637.

Nazratun Nafizah, A., et al. "Aqueous calyxes extract of Roselle or *Hibiscus sabdariffa* Linn supplementation improves liver morphology in streptozotocin induced diabetic rats." *Arab J. Gastroenterol*. 2017 Mar; 18(1): 13–20.

Inrahim, K., et al. "Erythrocyte osmotic fragility and general health status of adolescent Sprague Dawley rats supplemented with *Hibiscus sabdariffa* aqueous calyx extracts as neonates followed by a high-fructose diet post-weaning." *J. Anim. Physiol. Anim. Nutr*. 2018 Feb; 102(1): 114–121.

Peng, C., et al. "*Hibiscus sabdariffa* polyphenols alleviate insulin resistance and renal epithelial to mesenchymal transition: a novel action mechanism mediated by type 4 dipeptidyl peptidase." *J. Agric. Food Chem*. 2014 Oct; 62(40): 9736–43.

Wisetmuen, E., et al. "Insulin secretion enhancing activity of roselle calyx extract in normal and streptozotocin-induced diabetic rats." *Pharmacognosy Res*. 2013 Apr; 5(2): 65–70.

Idris, M., et al. "Protective role of *Hibiscus sabdariffa* calyx extract against streptozotocin induced sperm damage in diabetic rats." *EXCLI J*. 2012 Sep; 11: 659-66.

Diarrhea

Ali, M., et al. "Antinociceptive, anti-inflammatory and antidiarrheal activities of ethanolic calyx extract of *Hibiscus sabdariffa* Linn. (Malvaceae) in mice." *Zhong Xi Yi Jie He Xue Bao*. 2011 Jun; 9(6): 626-31.

References

Diuretic Actions

Nwachukwu, D., et al. "Does consumption of an aqueous extract of *Hibiscus sabdariffa* affect renal function in subjects with mild to moderate hypertension?" *J. Physiol. Sci.* 2017 Jan; 67(1): 227–234.

Jimenez-Ferrer, E., "Diuretic effect of compounds from *Hibiscus sabdariffa* by modulation of the aldosterone activity." *Planta Med.* 2012 Dec; 78(18): 1893–8.

Alarcon-Alonso, J., et al. "Pharmacological characterization of the diuretic effect of *Hibiscus sabdariffa* Linn (Malvaceae) extract." *J. Ethnopharmacol.* 2012 Feb; 139(3): 751–6.

Wright, C., et al. "Herbal medicines as diuretics: a review of the scientific evidence." *J. Ethnopharmacol.* 2007 Oct; 114(1): 1–31.

Karumi, Y., et al. "The protective effect of the aqueous extract of the calyx of *Hibiscus sabdariffa* roselle on the kidneys of salt-loaded rats." *J. Med. Lab. Sci.* 2003. 12(1): 46.

Heart-Protective Actions

Si, L., et al. "Roselle attenuates cardiac hypertrophy after myocardial infarction *in vivo* and *in vitro*." *EXCLI J.* 2019 Sep; 18: 876-892.

Abubarkar, S., et al. "Acute effects of *Hibiscus sabdariffa* calyces on postprandial blood pressure, vascular function, blood lipids, biomarkers of insulin resistance and inflammation in humans." *Nutrients*. 2019 Feb 5; 11(2): 341.

Perez-Torres, I., et al. "Myocardial protection from ischemia-reperfusion damage by the antioxidant effect of *Hibiscus sabdariffa* Linnaeus on metabolic syndrome rats." *Oxid. Med. Cell. Longev.* 2019 Mar 26; 2019: 1724194.

Ali, S., et al. "Anti-fibrotic actions of roselle extract in rat model of myocardial infarction." *Cardiovasc. Toxicol.* 2019 Feb; 19(1): 72–81.

Mohammed Yusof, N., et al. "*Hibiscus sabdariffa* (roselle) polyphenol-rich extract averts cardiac functional and structural abnormalities in type 1 diabetic rats." *Appl. Physiol. Nutr. Metab.* 2018 Dec; 43(12): 1224–1232.

Hosseini, A., et al. "Protective effect of *Hibiscus sabdariffa* on doxorubicin-induced cytotoxicity in H9c2 cardiomyoblast cells." *Iran J. Pharm. Res.* 2017 Spring; 16(2): 708–713.

Soto, M., et al. "Infusion of *Hibiscus sabdariffa* L. modulates oxidative stress in patients with Marfan Syndrome." *Mediators Inflamm.* 2016; 2016: 8625203.

Lim, Y., et al. "Roselle polyphenols exert potent negative inotropic effects via modulation of intracellular calcium regulatory channels in isolated rat heart." *Cardiovasc. Toxicol.* 2017 Jul; 17(3): 251–259.

Beltran-Debon, R., et al. "The acute impact of polyphenols from *Hibiscus sabdariffa* in metabolic homeostasis: an approach combining metabolomics and gene-expression analyses." *Food Funct.* 2015 Sep; 6(9): 2957–66.

Micucci, M., et al. "Cardiac and vascular synergic protective effect of *Olea europea* L. leaves and *Hibiscus sabdariffa* L. flower extracts." *Oxid. Med. Cell. Longev.* 2015; 2015: 318125.

Perez-Torres, I., et al. "Modification of the liver fatty acids by *Hibiscus sabdariffa* Linnaeus (Malvaceae) infusion, its possible effect on vascular reactivity in a metabolic syndrome model." *Clin. Exp. Hypertens.* 2014; 36(3): 123–31.

Inuwa, I., et al. "Long-term ingestion of *Hibiscus sabdariffa* calyx extract enhances myocardial capillarization in the spontaneously hypertensive rat." *Exp. Biol. Med.* 2012 May; 237(5): 563–9.

Huang, C., et al. "*Hibiscus sabdariffa* inhibits vascular smooth muscle cell proliferation and migration induced by high glucose-a mechanism involves connective tissue growth factor signals." *J. Agric. Food Chem.* 2009 Apr 22; 57(8): 3073–9.

Jonadet, M., et al. "*In vitro* enzyme inhibitory and *in vivo* cardioprotective activities of hibiscus (*Hibiscus sabdariffa* L.)]. *J. Pharm. Belg.* 1990 Mar–Apr; 45(2): 120–4.

Immunomodulatory Actions

Zheng, D., et al. "Purification, characterization and immunoregulatory activity of a polysaccharide isolated from *Hibiscus sabdariffa* L." *J. Sci. Food Agric.* 2017 Mar; 97(5): 1599–1606.

Fakeye, T., et al. "Immunomodulatory effect of extracts of *Hibiscus sabdariffa* L. (Family Malvaceae) in a mouse model." *Phytother. Res.* 2008 May; 22(5): 664–8.

Fakeye, T., et al. "Toxicity and immunomodulatory activity of fractions of *Hibiscus sabdariffa* Linn (family Malvaceae) in animal models." *Afr. J. Tradit. Complement. Altern. Med.* 2008 Jun; 5(4): 394–8.

References

Kidney-Protective Actions

Ali, B., et al. "Effect of aqueous extract and anthocyanins of calyces of *Hibiscus sabdariffa* (Malvaceae) in rats with adenine-induced chronic kidney disease." *J. Pharm. Pharmacol.* 2017 Sep; 69(9): 1219–1229.

Huang, C., et al. "*Hibiscus sabdariffa* polyphenols prevent palmitate-induced renal epithelial mesenchymal transition by alleviating dipeptidyl peptidase-4-mediated insulin resistance." *Food Funct.* 2016 Jan; 7(1): 475–82.

Anwar Ibrahim, D., et al. "Evaluation of the potential nephroprotective and antimicrobial effect of *Camellia sinensis* leaves versus *Hibiscus sabdariffa* (*in vivo* and *in vitro* studies)." *Adv. Pharmacol. Sci.* 2014; 2014: 389834.

Ademiluyi, A., et al. "Anthocyanin - rich red dye of *Hibiscus sabdariffa* calyx modulates cisplatin-induced nephrotoxicity and oxidative stress in rats." *Int. J. Biomed. Sci.* 2013 Dec; 9(4): 243–8.

Yang, Y., et al. "Polyphenols of *Hibiscus sabdariffa* improved diabetic nephropathy via attenuating renal epithelial mesenchymal transition." *J. Agric. Food Chem.* 2013 Aug; 61(31): 7545–51.

Seujange, Y., et al. "*Hibiscus sabdariffa* Linnaeus aqueous extracts attenuate the progression of renal injury in 5/6 nephrectomy rats." *Ren. Fail.* 2013; 35(1): 118–25.

Olatunji, L., et al. "Effects of aqueous extract of *Hibiscus sabdariffa* on renal Na(+)-K(+)-ATPase and Ca(2+)-Mg(2+)-ATPase activities in Wistar rats." *Zhong Xi Yi Jie He Xue Bao.* 2012 Sep; 10(9): 1049–55.

Wang, S., et al. "Aqueous extract from *Hibiscus sabdariffa* Linnaeus ameliorate diabetic nephropathy via regulating oxidative status and Akt/Bad/14-3-3γ in an experimental animal model." *Evid. Based Complement. Alternat. Med.* 2011; 2011: 938126.

Lee, W., et al. "Polyphenol extracts from *Hibiscus sabdariffa* Linnaeus attenuate nephropathy in experimental type 1 diabetes." *J. Agric. Food Chem.* 2009 Mar; 57(6): 2206–10.

Kidney Stone Prevention and Gout

Nirumand, M., et al. "Dietary plants for the prevention and management of kidney stones: preclinical and clinical evidence and molecular mechanisms." *Int. J. Mol. Sci.* 2018 Mar; 19(3): E765.

Hassan, S., et al. "Biological evaluation and molecular docking of protocatechuic acid from *Hibiscus sabdariffa* L. as a potent urease inhibitor by an ESI-MS based method." *Molecules*. 2017 Oct; 22(10): E1696.

Laikangbam, R., et al. "Inhibition of calcium oxalate crystal deposition on kidneys of urolithiatic rats by *Hibiscus sabdariffa* L. extract." *Urol. Res.* 2012 Jun; 40(3): 211–8.

Woottisin, S., et al. "Effects of *Orthosiphon grandiflorus, Hibiscus sabdariffa* and *Phyllanthus amarus* extracts on risk factors for urinary calcium oxalate stones in rats." *J. Urol.* 2011 Jan; 185(1): 323–8.

Prasongwatana, V., et al. "Uricosuric effect of Roselle (*Hibiscus sabdariffa*) in normal and renal-stone former subjects." *J. Ethnopharmacol.* 2008 May; 117(3): 491–5.

Kirdpon, S., et al. "Changes in urinary chemical composition in healthy volunteers after consuming roselle (*Hibiscus sabdariffa* Linn.) juice." *J. Med. Assoc .Thai.* 1994 Jun; 77(6): 314–21.

Liver-Protective Actions

Famurewa, A., et al. "Abrogation of hepatic damage induced by anticancer drug methotrexate by zobo (*Hibiscus sabdariffa* extract) supplementation via targeting oxidative hepatotoxicity in rats." *J. Diet. Suppl.* 2019; 16(3): 318–330.

Nazratun Nafizah, A., et al. "Aqueous calyxes extract of Roselle or *Hibiscus sabdariffa* Linn supplementation improves liver morphology in streptozotocin induced diabetic rats." *Arab J. Gastroenterol.* 2017 Mar; 18(1): 13–20.

Rodriguez-Ramiro, I., "Polyphenols and non-alcoholic fatty liver disease: impact and mechanisms." *Proc. Nutr. Soc.* 2016 Feb; 75(1): 47–60.

Adeyemi, D., et al. "Anti-hepatotoxic activities of *Hibiscus sabdariffa* L. in animal model of streptozotocin diabetes-induced liver damage." *BMC Complement. Altern. Med.* 2014 Jul 30; 14: 277.

Lee, C., et al. "A polyphenol extract of *Hibiscus sabdariffa* L. ameliorates acetaminophen-induced hepatic steatosis by attenuating the mitochondrial dysfunction *in vivo* and *in vitro*." *Biosci. Biotechnol. Biochem.* 2012; 76(4): 646–51.

Yin, G., et al. "Hepatoprotective and antioxidant effects of *Hibiscus sabdariffa* extract against carbon tetrachloride-induced hepatocyte damage in *Cyprinus carpio*." *In Vitro Cell. Dev. Biol. Anim.* 2011 Jan; 47(1): 10–5.

References

Liu, L., et al. "Aqueous extract of *Hibiscus sabdariffa* L. decelerates acetaminophen-induced acute liver damage by reducing cell death and oxidative stress in mouse experimental models." *J. Sci. Food Agric.* 2010 Jan; 90(2): 329–37.

Adaramoye, O., et al. "Protective effects of extracts of *Vernonia amygdalina*, *Hibiscus sabdariffa* and vitamin C against radiation-induced liver damage in rats." *J. Radiat. Res.* 2008 Mar; 49(2): 123–31.

Olaleye, M., et al. "Acetaminophen-induced liver damage in mice: effects of some medicinal plants on the oxidative defense system." *Exp. Toxicol. Pathol.* 2008 Mar; 59(5): 319–27.

Olalye, M., et al. "Commonly used tropical medicinal plants exhibit distinct *in vitro* antioxidant activities against hepatotoxins in rat liver." *Exp. Toxicol. Pathol.* 2007 Aug; 58(6): 433–8.

Liu, J., et al. "The protective effects of *Hibiscus sabdariffa* extract on CCl4-induced liver fibrosis in rats." *Food Chem. Toxicol.* 2006 Mar; 44(3): 336–43.

Amin, A., et al. "Hepatoprotective effects of *Hibiscus*, *Rosmarinus* and *Salvia* on azathioprine-induced toxicity in rats." *Life Sci.* 2005 Jun; 77(3): 266–78.

Ali, B., et al. "The effect of a water extract and anthocyanins of *Hibiscus sabdariffa* L. on paracetamol-induced hepatoxicity in rats." *Phytother Res.* 2003 Jan; 17(1): 56–9.

Lin, W., et al. "Hibiscus protocatechuic acid inhibits lipopolysaccharide-induced rat hepatic damage." *Arch. Toxicol.* 2003 Jan; 77(1): 42–7.

Liu, C., et al. "*In vivo* protective effect of protocatechuic acid on tert-butyl hydroperoxide-induced rat hepatotoxicity." *Food Chem. Toxicol.* 2002 May; 40(5): 635–41.

Wang, C., et al. "Protective effect of Hibiscus anthocyanins against tert-butyl hydroperoxide-induced hepatic toxicity in rats." *Food Chem. Toxicol.* 2000 May; 38(5): 411–6.

Tseng, T., et al. "Protective effects of dried flower extracts of *Hibiscus sabdariffa* L. against oxidative stress in rat primary hepatocytes." *Food Chem. Toxicol.* 1997 Dec; 35(12): 1159–64.

Tseng, T., et al. "Hibiscus protocatechuic acid protects against oxidative damage induced by tert-butylhydroperoxide in rat primary hepatocytes." *Chem. Biol. Interact.* 1996 Aug; 101(2): 137–48.

111

Macular Degeneration

Joshua, M., et al. "Disruption of angiogenesis by anthocyanin-rich extracts of *Hibiscus sabdariffa*." *Int. J. Sci. Eng. Res.* 2017 Feb; 8(2): 299-307.

Memory and Cognitive Enhancement Actions

Bayani, G., et al. "Anti-inflammatory effects of *Hibiscus sabdariffa* Linn. on the IL-1β/IL-1ra ratio in plasma and hippocampus of overtrained rats and correlation with spatial memory." *Kobe J. Med. Sci.* 2018 Oct; 64(2): E73–E83.

Seung, T., et al. "Ethyl acetate fraction from *Hibiscus sabdariffa* L. attenuates diabetes-associated cognitive impairment in mice." *Food Res. Int.* 2018 Mar; 105: 589–598.

Metabolic Syndrome

Diez-Echava, P., et al. "The prebiotic properties of *Hibiscus sabdariffa* extract contribute to the beneficial effects in diet-induced obesity in mice." *Food Res. Int.* 2020 Jan; 127: 108722.

Zhang, B., et al. "Effect of *Hibiscus sabdariffa* (Roselle) supplementation in regulating blood lipids among patients with metabolic syndrome and related disorders: A systematic review and meta-analysis." *Phytother. Res.* 2019 Dec 12. (Ahead of print]

Ajoboye, T., et al. "*Hibiscus sabdariffa* calyx palliates insulin resistance, hyperglycemia, dyslipidemia and oxidative rout in fructose-induced metabolic syndrome rats." *J. Sci. Food Agric.* 2016 Mar; 96(5): 1522–31.

Perez-Torres, I., et al. "Modification of the liver fatty acids by *Hibiscus sabdariffa* Linnaeus (Malvaceae) infusion, its possible effect on vascular reactivity in a metabolic syndrome model." *Clin. Exp. Hypertens.* 2014; 36(3): 123-31.

Perez-Torres, I., et al. "*Hibiscus sabdariffa* Linnaeus (Malvaceae), curcumin and resveratrol as alternative medicinal agents against metabolic syndrome." *Cardiovasc. Hematol. Agents Med. Chem.* 2013 Mar; 11(1): 25–37.

Peng, C., et al. "*Hibiscus sabdariffa* polyphenolic extract inhibits hyperglycemia, hyperlipidemia, and glycation-oxidative stress while improving insulin resistance." *J. Agric. Food Chem.* 2011 Sep 28; 59(18): 9901–9.

Gurrola-Diaz, C., et al. "Effects of *Hibiscus sabdariffa* extract powder and preventive treatment (diet) on the lipid profiles of patients with metabolic syndrome (MeSy)." *Phytomedicine*. 2010 Jun; 17(7): 500–5.

References

Sedative and Anti-Anxiety Actions

Fakeye, T., et al. "Anxiolytic and sedative effects of extracts of *Hibiscus sabdariffa* Linn (family Malvaceae)." *Afr. J. Med. Med. Sci.* 2008 Mar; 37(1): 49–54.

UV-Protectant Actions

Ozkol, H., et al. "Anthocyanin-rich extract from *Hibiscus sabdariffa* calyx counteracts UVC-caused impairments in rats." *Pharm. Biol.* 2015; 53(10): 1435-41.

Review Articles

Riaz, G., et al. "A review on phytochemistry and therapeutic uses of *Hibiscus sabdariffa* L." *Biomed. Pharmacother.* 2018 Jun; 102: 575–586.

Olivares-Vicente, M., et al. "Plant-derived polyphenols in human health: biological activity, metabolites and putative molecular targets." *Curr. Drug. Metab.* 2018; 19(4): 351–369.

Abat, J., et al. "Ethnomedicinal, phytochemical and ethnopharmacological aspects of four medicinal plants of Malvaceae used in Indian traditional medicines: A review." *Medicines.* 2017 Oct 18; 4(4): E75.

Hassan, S., et al. "Antimicrobial, antiparasitic and anticancer properties of *Hibiscus sabdariffa* (L.) and its phytochemicals: *in vitro* and *in vivo* studies." *Ceska. Slov. Farm.* Winter 2016; 65(1): 10--4.

Serban, C., et al. "Effect of sour tea (*Hibiscus sabdariffa* L.) on arterial hypertension: a systematic review and meta-analysis of randomized controlled trials." *J. Hypertens.* 2015 Jun; 33(6): 1119--27.

Da-Costa-Rocha, I., et al. "*Hibiscus sabdariffa* L. - a phytochemical and pharmacological review." *Food Chem.* 2014 Dec; 165: 424–43.

Guardiola, S., et al. "[Therapeutic potential of *Hibiscus sabdariffa*: a review of the scientific evidence]." *Endocrinol. Nutr.* 2014 May; 61(5): 274–95.

Aziz, Z., et al. "Effects of *Hibiscus sabdariffa* L. on serum lipids: a systematic review and meta-analysis." *J. Ethnopharmacol.* 2013 Nov; 150(2): 442–50.

Carvajal-Zarrabal, O., et al. "*Hibiscus sabdariffa* L., roselle calyx, from ethnobotany to pharmacology." *J. Exp. Pharmacol.* 2012 Feb; 4: 25–39.

Wahabi, H., et al. "The effectiveness of *Hibiscus sabdariffa* in the treatment of hypertension: a systematic review." *Phytomedicine.* 2010 Feb; 17(2): 83–6.

Ali, B., et al. "Phytochemical, pharmacological and toxicological aspects of *Hibiscus sabdariffa* L.: a review." *Phytother. Res.* 2005 May; 19(5): 369–75.

Toxicity, Safety, and Drug Interaction Studies

Showande, J., et al. "*In vitro* modulation of cytochrome P450 isozymes and pharmacokinetics of caffeine by extracts of *Hibiscus sabdariffa* Linn calyx." *J. Basic Clin. Physiol. Pharmacol.* 2019 Apr; 30(3): 0206.

Peter, E., et al. "Efficacy of standardized extract of *Hibiscus sabdariffa* L. (Malvaceae) in improving iron status of adults in malaria endemic area: A randomized controlled trial." *J. Ethnopharmacol.* 2017 Sep; 209: 288–293.

Passaro, M., et al. "Effect of a food supplement containing l-methionine on urinary tract infections in pregnancy: a prospective, multicenter observational study." *J. Altern. Complement.* Med. 2017 Jun; 23(6): 471–478.

Schulzki, G., et al. "Transition rates of selected metals determined in various types of teas (*Camellia sinensis* L. Kuntze) and herbal/fruit infusions." *Food Chem.* 2017 Jan; 215: 22–30.

de Arruda, A., et al. "Safety assessment of *Hibiscus sabdariffa* after maternal exposure on male reproductive parameters in rats." *Drug Chem. Toxicol.* 2016; 39(1): 22–7.

Adenkola, A., et al. "Erythrocyte osmotic fragility and excitability score in rabbit fed *Hibiscus sabdariffa* in graded level." *Niger. J. Physiol. Sci.* 2014 Dec; 29(2): 113–7.

Sireeratawong, S., et al. "Toxicity studies of the water extract from the calyces of *Hibiscus sabdariffa* L. in rats." *Afr. J. Tradit. Complement. Altern. Med.* 2013 May; 10(4): 122–7.

Johnson, S., et al. "*In vitro* inhibitory activities of the extract of *Hibiscus sabdariffa* L. (family Malvaceae) on selected cytochrome P450 isoforms." *Afr. J. Tradit. Complement. Altern. Med.* 2013 Apr; 10(3): 533–40.

Ali, B., et al. "Effect of *Hibiscus sabdariffa* and its anthocyanins on some reproductive aspects in rats." *Nat. Prod. Commun.* 2012 Jan; 7(1): 41–4.

Mahmoud. Y. "Effect of extract of Hibiscus on the ultrastructure of the testis in adult mice." *Acta Histochem.* 2012 Jul; 114(4): 342–8.

Ndu, O., et al. "Herb-drug interaction between the extract of *Hibiscus*

References

sabdariffa L. and hydrochlorothiazide in experimental animals." *J. Med. Food*. 2011 Jun; 14(6): 640–4.

Iyare, E., et al. "Mechanism of delayed puberty in rats whose mothers consumed *Hibiscus sabdariffa* during lactation." *Pharm. Biol*. 2010 Oct; 48(10): 1170–6.

Iyare, E., et al. "Delayed puberty onset in rats that consumed aqueous extract of *Hibiscus sabdariffa* during the juvenile-pubertal period." *Pak. J. Biol. Sci*. 2009 Dec; 12(23): 1505–10.

Fakeye, T., et al. "Toxic effects of oral administration of extracts of dried calyx of *Hibiscus sabdariffa* Linn. (Malvaceae). *Phytother. Res*. 2009 Mar; 23(3): 412–6.

Fakeye, T., et al. "Effects of water extract of *Hibiscus sabdariffa*, Linn (Malvaceae) 'Roselle' on excretion of a diclofenac formulation." *Phytother. Res*. 2007 Jan; 21(1): 96–8.

Kolawole, J., "Effect of zobo drink (*Hibiscus sabdariffa* water extract) on the pharmacokinetics of acetaminophen in human volunteers." *Eur. J. Drug. Metab. Pharmacokinet*. 2004 Jan–Mar; 29(1): 25–9.

Orisakwe, O., et al. "Testicular effects of sub-chronic administration of *Hibiscus sabdariffa* calyx aqueous extract in rats." *Reprod. Toxicol*. 2004 Mar–Apr; 18(2): 295–8.

Akindahunsi, A., "Toxicological investigation of aqueous-methanolic extract of the calyces of *Hibiscus sabdariffa* L." *J. Ethnopharmacol*. 2003 Nov; 89(1): 161–4.

Chemical Constituents & Absorption

Długaszek, M., et al. "Assessment of the nutritional value of various teas infusions in terms of the macro- and trace elements content." *J. Trace Elem. Med. Biol*. 2019 Nov 4: 126428. (ahead of print)

Avalos-Martínez, E., et al. "Assessment of volatile compounds and sensory characteristics of Mexican hibiscus (*Hibiscus sabdariffa* L.) calyces hot beverages." *J. Food Sci. Technol*. 2019 Jan; 56(1): 360–366.

Zheoat, A., et al. "Crystal structures of hibiscus acid and hibiscus acid dimethyl ester isolated from *Hibiscus sabdariffa* (Malvaceae)." *Acta Crystallogr. E. Crystallogr. Commun*. 2017 Aug; 73(Pt 9): 1368–1371.

Grajeda-Iglesias, C., "Isolation and characterization of anthocyanins from *Hibiscus sabdariffa* flowers." *J. Nat. Prod*. 2016 Jul 22; 79(7): 1709–18.

Ifie, I., et al. "*Hibiscus sabdariffa* (Roselle) extracts and wine: phytochemical profile, physicochemical properties, and carbohydrase inhibition." *J. Agric. Food Chem.* 2016 Jun; 64(24): 4921–31.

Vidot, K., et al. "Effect of temperature on acidity and hydration equilibrium constants of delphinidin-3-o- and cyanidin-3-o-sambubioside calculated from uni- and multiwavelength spectroscopic data." *J. Agric. Food Chem.* 2016 May 25; 64(20): 4139–45.

Farag, M., et al. "Volatiles and primary metabolites profiling in two *Hibiscus sabdariffa* (roselle) cultivars via headspace SPME-GC-MS and chemometrics." *Food Res. Int.* 2015 Dec; 78: 327–-335.

Borras-Linares, I., et al. "Permeability study of polyphenols derived from a phenolic-enriched *Hibiscus sabdariffa* extract by UHPLC-ESI-UHR-Qq-TOF-MS." *Int. J. Mol. Sci.* 2015 Aug; 16(8): 18396–411.

Cahlikova, L., et al. "Anthocyanins of *Hibiscus sabdariffa* calyces from Sudan." *Nat. Prod. Commun.* 2015 Jan; 10(1): 77–9.

Sindi, H., et al. "Comparative chemical and biochemical analysis of extracts of *Hibiscus sabdariffa*." *Food Chem.* 2014 Dec; 164: 23–9.

Camelo-Méndez, G., et al. "Comparative study of anthocyanin and volatile compounds content of four varieties of Mexican roselle (*Hibiscus sabdariffa* L.) by multivariable analysis." *Plant Foods Hum. Nutr. 2013* Sep; 68(3): 229–34.

Ramirez-Rodrigues, M., et al. "Physicochemical and phytochemical properties of cold and hot water extraction from *Hibiscus sabdariffa*." *J. Food Sci.* 2011 Apr; 76(3): C428-35.

Sayago-Ayerdi, S., et al. "[Hibiscus sabdariffa L: source of antioxidant dietary fiber]." *Arch. Latinoam. Nutr.* 2010 Mar; 60(1): 79–84.

Rodríguez-Medina, I., et al. "Direct characterization of aqueous extract of *Hibiscus sabdariffa* using HPLC with diode array detection coupled to ESI and ion trap MS." *J. Sep. Sci.* 2009 Oct; 32(20): 3441–8.

Segura-Carretero, A., "Selective extraction, separation, and identification of anthocyanins from *Hibiscus sabdariffa* L. using solid phase extraction-capillary electrophoresis-mass spectrometry (time-of-flight / ion trap)." *Electrophoresis.* 2008 Jul; 29(13): 2852–61.

Muller, B., et al. "Chemical structure and biological activity of polysaccharides from *Hibiscus sabdariffa*." *Planta Med.* 1992 Feb; 58(1): 60–7.

References

Manufacturing & Quality Control

Deli, M., et al. "Successive grinding and sieving as a new tool to fractionate polyphenols and antioxidants of plants powders: Application to *Boscia senegalensis* seeds, *Dichrostachys glomerata* fruits, and *Hibiscus sabdariffa* calyx powders." *Food Sci. Nutr.* 2019 Apr; 7(5): 1795–1806.

Gomez-Aldapa, C., et al. "A modified Achira (*Canna indica* L.) starch as a wall material for the encapsulation of *Hibiscus sabdariffa* extract using spray drying." *Food Res. Int.* 2019 May; 119: 547–553.

Pinela, J., et al. "Optimization of heat- and ultrasound-assisted extraction of anthocyanins from *Hibiscus sabdariffa* calyces for natural food colorants." *Food Chem.* 2019 Mar; 275: 309–321.

Achir, N., et al. "Monitoring anthocyanin degradation in *Hibiscus sabdariffa* extracts with multi-curve resolution on spectral measurement during storage." *Food Chem.* 2019 Jan; 271: 536–542.

Juhari, N., et al. "Characterization of roselle calyx from different geographical origins." *Food Res. Int.* 2018 Oct; 112: 378–389.

Djaeni, M., et al. "Drying rate and product quality evaluation of roselle (*Hibiscus sabdariffa* L.) calyces extract dried with foaming agent under different temperatures." *Int. J. Food Sci.* 2018 Mar 20; 2018: 9243549.

Ifie, I., et al. "Seasonal variation in *Hibiscus sabdariffa* (Roselle) calyx phytochemical profile, soluble solids and α-glucosidase inhibition." *Food Chem.* 2018 Sep; 261: 164–168.

Pimentel-Moral, S., et al. "Microwave-assisted extraction for *Hibiscus sabdariffa* bioactive compounds." *J. Pharm. Biomed. Anal.* 2018 Jul; 156: 313–322.

Liu, X., et al. "Development of an ultrasonication-assisted extraction based HPLC with a fluorescence method for sensitive determination of aflatoxins in highly acidic *Hibiscus sabdariffa*." *Front. Pharmacol.* 2018 Apr 6; 9: 284.

Nguyen, T., et al. "Encapsulation of *Hibiscus sabdariffa* L. anthocyanins as natural colours in yeast." *Food Res. Int.* 2018 May; 107: 275–280.

Juhari, N., et al. "Physicochemical properties and oxidative storage stability of milled roselle *(Hibiscus sabdariffa* L.) seeds." *Molecules.* 2018 Feb; 23(2): E385.

de Moura S., et al. "Encapsulating anthocyanins from *Hibiscus sabdariffa* L. calyces by ionic gelation: Pigment stability during storage of microparticles." *Food Chem.* 2018 Feb; 241: 317–327.

Ochoa-Velasco C., et al. "Antioxidant characteristics of extracts of *Hibiscus sabdariffa* calyces encapsulated with mesquite gum." *J. Food Sci. Technol.* 2017 Jun; 54(7): 1747–1756.

Sinela, A., et al. "Anthocyanins degradation during storage of *Hibiscus sabdariffa* extract and evolution of its degradation products." Food Chem. 2017 Jan; 214: 234–241.

Sinela, A., et al. "Exploration of reaction mechanisms of anthocyanin degradation in a roselle extract through kinetic studies on formulated model media." *Food Chem.* 2017 Nov; 235: 67–75.

Opletala, L., et al. "Preparation and validated analysis of anthocyanin concentrate from the calyces of *Hibiscus sabdariffa*." *Nat. Prod. Commun.* 2017 Jan; 12(1): 43–45.

Camelo-Méndez, G., "Comparative study of phenolic profile, antioxidant capacity, and color-composition relation of roselle cultivars with contrasting pigmentation." *Plant Foods Hum. Nutr.* 2016 Mar; 71(1): 109–14.

Badejo, A., et al. "Processing effects on the antioxidant activities of beverage blends developed from *Cyperus esculentus*, *Hibiscus sabdariffa*, and *Moringa oleifera* extracts." *Prev. Nutr. Food Sci.* 2014 Sep; 19(3): 227–33.

Sáyago-Ayerdi. S., et al. "By-product from decoction process of *Hibiscus sabdariffa* L. calyces as a source of polyphenols and dietary fiber." *J. Sci. Food Agric.* 2014 Mar; 94(5): 898–904.

Cisse, M., et al. "Impact of the extraction procedure on the kinetics of anthocyanin and colour degradation of roselle extracts during storage." *J. Sci. Food Agric.* 2012 Apr; 92(6): 1214–21.

Gonzalez-Palomares, S., et al. "Effect of the temperature on the spray drying of Roselle extracts (*Hibiscus sabdariffa* L.)." *Plant Foods Hum. Nutr.* 2009 Mar; 64(1): 62–7.

Marco, P., et al. "Exploratory analysis of simultaneous degradation of anthocyanins in the calyces of flowers of the *Hibiscus sabdariffa* species by PARAFAC model." *Anal. Sci.* 2005 Dec; 21(12): 1523–7.

About the Author

Leslie Taylor is one of the world's leading experts on rainforest medicinal plants. She founded, managed, and directed the Raintree group of companies from 1995 to 2012, and was a leader in creating a worldwide market for the important medicinal plants of the Amazon rainforest.

Having survived a rare form of leukemia only because of alternative health and herbal medicine, Leslie has been researching, studying, and documenting alternative healing modalities—including herbal medicine—for more than thirty years. A dedicated herbalist and naturopath, she developed many herbal formulas and remedies for her companies, for practitioners, and for individuals needing help. In 1995, while researching alternative AIDS and cancer therapies in Europe, Leslie became aware of a medicinal plant from the Peruvian rainforest called cat's claw. This research took her to the Peruvian rainforest to gain firsthand knowledge about this new medicinal plant. Upon her return, she founded Raintree Nutrition, Inc., to make this important rainforest medicinal plant and others available in the United States.

After that first trip, Leslie returned to the Amazon numerous times, continuing to research and document more rainforest medicinal plants. In these endeavors, she worked directly with indigenous Indian shamans and healers, learning about their use of healing plants, as well as with indigenous tribal communities and other rainforest communities. She also worked with phytochemists, botanists, ethnobotanists, researchers, and alternative and integrative health practitioners to document, research, test, and validate rainforest medicinal plants.

In 2012, with many other companies selling the rainforest plants that she had introduced to the United States, she decided to close her business and naturopathic practice and devote herself to educating people about the benefits of medicinal plants. She freely shared all her proprietary formulas by posting them on the Raintree website so that anyone can make and use them.

Now, Leslie Taylor remains a trusted source of factual information about rainforest medicinal plants and continues to update the Tropical Plant Database for these purposes. A practicing board certified naturopath for many years (now retired), she has lectured and taught classes in naturopathic medicine, herbal medicine, and ethnobotany, as well as environmental and sustainability issues in the Amazon rainforest. She is the author of *Herbal Secrets of the Rainforest* and of the best-selling *The Healing Power of Rainforest Herbs,* as well as the highly popular and extensively referenced Raintree Tropical Plant Database (http://www.rain-tree.com/plants.htm), which has been online since 1996.

More information about Leslie Taylor and her other books can be found at http://rain-tree.com/author.htm and on her Amazon Author Page. She also has a personal blog where you can ask questions and share your results using hibiscus flowers and other heart-healthy strategies with others at http://leslie-taylor-raintree.blogspot.com/hibiscus-flower.html.

www.ingramcontent.com/pod-product-compliance
Lightning Source LLC
Chambersburg PA
CBHW050735030426
42336CB00012B/1572